Bulletproof Entrepreneur

How To Stay Fit and Healthy While Running Your Business

Paul N Miller

RETHINK PRESS

First published in Great Britain 2015 by Rethink Press (www.rethinkpress.com)

© Copyright Paul N Miller

All rights reserved. No part of this publication may be reproduced, stored in or introduced into a retrieval system, or transmitted, in any form, or by any means (electronic, mechanical, photocopying, recording or otherwise) without the prior written permission of the publisher.

The right of Paul N Miller to be identified as the author of this work has been asserted by him in accordance with the Copyright, Designs and Patents Act 1988.

This book is sold subject to the condition that it shall not, by way of trade or otherwise, be lent, resold, hired out, or otherwise circulated without the publisher's prior consent in any form of binding or cover other than that in which it is published and without a similar condition including this condition being imposed on the subsequent purchaser.

Cover image © www.shutterstock.com

Contents

Foreword	1
Introduction	5
ONE - My Story	9
TWO - What Is Success	19
THREE - Step One - Meaning	29
FOUR - Step Two - Movement	39
FIVE - Step Three - Mindful Meals	53
SIX - Step Four - Managing (Time and Stress)	65
SEVEN - Step Five - Madness	79
EIGHT - Bring It All Together	91
NINE - The Application	121
TEN - Young At Heart	131
Acknowledgments	141
Testimonials	143
The Author	146

Foreword

My path crossed Paul's at a mutual friend's book launch. Having worked with so many people, I knew in the first five minutes of our conversation that he was different from the many Personal Trainers that I have coached. His soul was searching for a teacher to help him navigate through the noise, the fears, and the distractions that prevented him from living his true values, being creative, and freeing his soul from the self-made inner prison.

After his initial consultation he committed to the 'Love Your Life, Live Your Dreams' yearly Integrated Coaching Program. Through every coaching session we had, Paul was committed, consistent, and eager to get to the root cause of every life adversity he had ever had. With time passing I saw him free himself from the many limiting beliefs, fears, and conditioning that held him back from truly honouring his personal values. The deeper he went within, the more he dug out un-resourceful parts of his consciousness, the closer he got to his own treasure chest that was buried underneath a hurdle of life adversities. The wider his perception of who he really is became, the louder his heart's authentic voice started to be.

It is this free voice that comes from the depth of his being that I now read and recognise in every word of *Bulletproof Entrepreneur*. Having witnessed personally Paul's shifts in consciousness, ways of thinking, being, and expanding his capacity to love, I knew that this book would be exceptional. He once again hit a home run for the conscious entrepreneurs' movement. Read this book with a childlike curiosity and you will make your entrepreneurial journey so much more enjoyable, fun and fulfilling.

In this book, Paul takes you on a journey that highlights the many challenges of being an entrepreneur. You will come across many compelling discoveries that awaken us to the truth of how easily many entrepreneurs can end up working long hours, feeling lonely, and becoming socially isolated.

In every sphere of our busy lives we are robbed of one very important thing: time. Through his personal adventures and many of his clients' stories, Paul's book shows us practical tools that we can use as entrepreneurs to save time, be healthier, and look after our physical and emotional wellbeing.

Paul has taken his years of experience working as a Personal Trainer in the wellness industry, studying and training other Personal Trainers, combined with his depth of spiritual perception, and turned these into a simple, five-step method and a must have manual that helps us become conscious, fun and healthy *Bulletproof Entrepreneurs*.

Whether you are an entrepreneur or aspiring to be one, this book provides a prescription for creating and strengthening the habits that are essential to improving your wealth through movement, fun and maintaining great health.

He has captured the deceptive nature of our Entrepreneurial Ego, and introduced it in such a succinct and sophisticated manner as to leave the reader fully empowered to take the reins of their life and start taking back control.

Use his 90-day formula, commit to it, and see how each passing day you too can come a step closer to happiness and the success that if you give yourself permission you too can achieve and have. Each chapter in this book has lessons learned, stories, case studies and practical exercises that will help you recognise and understand what stops you from being a happy, wealthy and inspired entrepreneur.

But this timely and important book is much more than a description of the problems that many entrepreneurs face; it is your key to unlocking your inner child that loves fun, exploring and learning to be free.

If, like me, you have spent a lifetime in the gym and long hours building your business, and now realise that your time is your most precious commodity, then you will find reading Paul's book an enriching and rewarding experience.

Tony J Selimi
Business Success Coach, Keynote Speaker, Best-selling Author.

Introduction

Welcome to the new world of business ownership. A way of life that enables you to work less and live more. A guide to help you preserve your health for the long term, achieve great success and enjoy each and every day.

I have come to realise that the more we work, the more we distance ourselves from each other, from our social network and, more importantly, from true health and vitality. We are neglecting what we truly want from life for the sake of working hard. I believe that working hard is an old-school approach to life that no longer works.

In my time in the health and fitness industry, I have met so many people who try to fit all the "health stuff" in little snippets of time around running their business and often end up neglecting things altogether. What these people have failed to realise is the negative effects this could have on them in the long term, with regard to potential injury and illness.

In this book I will share with you what I believe are the keys to success and how to obtain it. By following my approach you will be able to work less, have more fun and recapture that energy and vitality from your youth. This is not a book that will give you quick and easy ways to exercise and eat well, if you get a chance, in your busy day. If anything, this is a book that will teach you how to fit quick and easy ways of working around your busy day of living!

The constant chase for financial success has the potential to open up a world of poor health and suffering. We find ourselves working long hours and as a result we become stressed. This stress then forces us to make poor food choices, for example, that give us instant satisfaction. Our energy levels start to deplete and we feel too tired to go and exercise. The lack of exercise drops our energy levels even further and we lose productivity in our work. Now begins a vicious circle of constantly chasing those elusive energy levels.

What I have found is that we have become fixated on the future. We have come to think that the answer to everything is to get our heads down for a number of years and we will then be able to sell up and be free. What we have not realised, until now, is that this rarely ever happens to people, and if it does, they will have sacrificed so much to get there. I understand the importance of sacrifice but I believe there is a limit.

We work so much that we neglect our social life and may find ourselves having a few too many drinks at the weekend to help us "unwind". Monday hits and we feel a little worse for wear. To top this off, while we drink ourselves silly we are constantly complaining about how tough life is. Over time, we find ourselves out of shape and even lower in energy.

You will learn about why you are so concerned with working every hour under the sun; what effects that has on not only your physical wellbeing but also your mental and emotional wellbeing; and how to create a balance in your life that enables you to make the most of *now*. You will learn the importance of stress and time management, not to mention exercise and nutrition. I also go over how important fun and social interaction are for us.

Using case studies of clients, interviews with entrepreneurs and my own personal experiences, I have highlighted the importance of putting yourself and your health among your top priorities. I believe this is the key to being more productive in work and enjoying a better, more adventurous life.

This book is for the entrepreneurs and business owners out there who are serious about getting the most out of life, with optimal health and vitality, without losing focus on their business. I believe that with the strategies I will talk through in this book, you will find that your focus sharpens up even more and takes you to a point of greater business success.

Life really is far too short to be spending it getting worked up over little things that deep down really do not matter. It is also far too short to just let fly by without making the most of it. We have access to a world of abundance right at our fingertips and yet we spend most of our waking hours toiling away at project after project that takes us far longer to complete than it ought to.

We became entrepreneurs for a reason. We have a desire to solve problems. We refuse to work for anyone else and we want to be in control of our own destiny. So why is it that we start to lose control of everything of real importance when busy times come along? Why can we not just enjoy the best of all worlds?

My aim is to help create more fun and fulfilment in the world. I believe that this will drastically reduce illness and disease. Apart from ourselves there is nothing stopping us having this life now. We just need to decide what it is that we value the most and start living in congruence with these values.

All I want is to do more and experience more of what life has to offer. It is difficult to do that when we are all at work. We have 24 hours in a day so why is it that when we are not sleeping we are either working or too tired to do anything? Why are we just OK with missing out on new things for the sake of work? Why have we not yet managed to get that balance right?

Nothing I tell you in this book is anything you do not already know. All I will be doing is helping you raise your conscious awareness of your current behaviours to help improve the quality of your life. A very high percentage of small businesses fail in the early stages or struggle for many years. Live the life you want to live and you will be sure to be in the minority.

ONE
My Story

"Honesty and openness is always the foundation of insightful dialogue."
BELL HOOKS

There I was, walking to the man-made beach in Brisbane with my friends Hannah and Rachel. For some reason we brought up the subject of careers. Hannah is an osteopath and Rachel is a nurse. They had studied for qualifications and had their careers mapped out. As soon as they got home, they were sorted.

Until I went to Australia I had only ever done office work such as banking and accounting. I remember saying that day that I had no clue what I was going to do when I got back home but whatever it would be, I would put my all in and work as hard as I possibly could to succeed. Looking back now, that was by far the dumbest thing I have ever said!

I have always prided myself on working hard, whatever I do. Once I get into the flow of things I devote myself to it and always do well. For example, in Australia I got a job in a bar. I had never done bar work in my life – which was pretty obvious at the time – but I stuck with it. I was dedicated and hungry. Within seven months I was running the place.

Going to Australia in the first place was a chance for me to escape the daily routine of London life and just chill out and have some fun. I never thought I would be there as long as I was, but in fact I only really enjoyed the first year of the two I spent there. Before long I was submerged in the seriousness of working life again. You would have thought that working behind a bar in Australia would have been a great deal of fun. Do not get me wrong, it certainly had its perks, but trust me to take my work so seriously!

Fast forward 18 months from that day in Brisbane and my Australian visa was due for expiry. I felt the time had come to head back to Blighty and really make something of myself. I had decided on a career in Personal Training and went in all guns blazing. I enrolled on the course before I even left Australia and could not wait to get home so that I could start. I landed on the Thursday and started my course on the following Monday.

My reasons for wanting to get into the fitness industry were pretty simple. I did not want to go back to office work; I would run my own diary and I could wear a pair of shorts every day if I wanted to. This was the perfect job for me as it would give me the flexibility and freedom I desired. Or so I thought.

Now I am a business owner. I am responsible for making my own living. I do not have the "safety" of a job where I would still be getting paid the same at the end of the month. I have to go out and make my own living as well as keeping on top of all the admin stuff such as keeping accounts, and designing client programmes. Not only that, my industry requires constant study.

Nothing had prepared me for what this new industry had in store. It is a tough gig, with long exhausting hours, long periods of loneliness and really bad pay when operating through a commercial gym. There have been several times when I wanted to quit and just find something else, but I kept at it in the hope that one day I would get my just rewards and have the life I wanted.

Having a job can be tough and often requires more than the 35-40 hours that you are contracted for. Having a business is a full contact sport. It always requires a lot more than the 60-80 hours we actually end up working. It makes us give our blood, sweat and tears.

This was the choice I made, though, and I am too stubborn to quit anything so I decided to suck it up and get on with it. I set about bringing in the clients I needed and got to work. Despite an incredibly tough first year, I started to get into my flow from year two and built up a vast experience of delivering personal training sessions in high volume.

It took me a while to figure it out, but I started to see a common trend in my clients, most of whom are males in their late 30s to early 40s. Many were business owners, entrepreneurs or were responsible for generating their own income. They had such hectic schedules that in a lot of cases our sessions only lasted 45 minutes. They lived on quick and easy meals, regardless of nutritious content. Not to mention, they were stressed.

I found it bizarre that despite vast improvements they made with me, if something came up in their business then that would take priority and they would find it very easy to skip the stuff I advised outside our sessions together. I know that accountability is key and with someone standing over you, you push yourself that bit harder, but I just did not understand why their health seemed to play second fiddle. Especially if they are responsible for their own income.

As a Personal Trainer, I naturally study a lot about nutrition and exercise. Given that virtually everyone who comes to me has some kind of injury, I find myself getting more and more involved in learning about rehabilitation techniques. In a lot of cases these issues are very easily dealt with, and combined with better eating my clients are able to get some great results. What I could not understand was that there never seemed to be any desire to really maximise these gains and seek the optimal vitality we are all capable of.

My Story

Before I knew it, I was in the exact same position. I found myself experiencing this world of putting work before everything else again. I was helping so many people improve their health and fitness levels that I was completely neglecting my own. I was working 12-15 hour days, often with several back-to-back sessions, and trying to grab the odd nap wherever I could just so I could see out the day with at least a glimmer of energy.

My training went completely by the wayside. I went almost three months without doing a single training session because I was so drained and, quite frankly, I just could not be bothered. Not only that, I found myself constantly pigging out on junk food. Quite shocking for someone working in health and fitness, I know!

In fact, every evening I got to Charing Cross station I would pick up a few chocolate bars or biscuits. I needed something, anything, to give me a hit of gratification and make me feel good, albeit temporarily. I even confess to one or two occasions going into McDonalds first thing in the morning for breakfast, right before a 7am client, because I was so tired and it made me feel good. Albeit temporarily, again!

I started to dig deeper to try to understand why we find ourselves so immersed in our work that nothing else matters. Sure, a lot of us are fortunate enough to enjoy what we do, but I do not believe that anything is worth sacrificing our health and our overall wellbeing for.

I just wanted to experience more from life: to do more things and have more holidays; to buy nice things; have a great social life with my friends and just have more fun. Then it just hit me. Like a ton of bricks. Working hard does not work.

It was starting to appear very obvious to me that I could work myself into the ground and in years to come I could be well off and financially secure. On the other side of the coin, though, I could also put everything into developing my health and become almost invincible. The fact was that I could not do both. It was impossible. I do believe we can *have* both, however.

To me, health is not just about fitness levels and eating right. It goes so much deeper than that. Health is a state of mind that thrives on many important factors such as fun, social interaction and relaxation. I had removed all of this from my life in the hope that if I worked my fingers to the bone for a few years then I would make it rich and then do what I wanted, knowing that I would have the financial independence to allow me to do this. I was chasing a life of freedom by going solely down the route of making money.

It became very clear to me sooner rather than later that this approach just does not work. Looking at my clients who had over 10 years of living in this manner taught me a very valuable lesson. Is this where I really wanted to get? Did I want to sacrifice everything I had had up until now to find myself working long hours and missing out on everything?

Where would they want to be in another 10 years? Where would they be if they carried on as they were? Was all this stress and pressure to succeed really worth it, especially if we go by the old school definition of success?

Going back to my bar job example, it was all well and good working my way up like that and giving it everything I had. However, what I did not realise at the time was that one by one, all my friends were heading off to other places to continue their travel. I also ended up alienating my girlfriend at the time. I missed out on doing so much great stuff. All because of work.

I have since learned that the definition of success is fulfilment. And to be fulfilled involves being the person I want to be and living my life the way I want to live it. To do the things I want to do wherever and whenever I like. I believe that life is there to be lived not just to exist and accept things we disagree with.

Living, for me, involves honouring my values. Always chasing money is not necessarily going to help me honour my values. By knowing what my core values are and being congruent with them and not subordinating to anyone else's, means I can live the life I truly want. And what I truly want is to squeeze more juice out of the fruit. So to speak.

Making this discovery has been the biggest game-changer for me. By knowing that my core values are health, fun, learning, teaching, and, of course, money, I have developed a lifestyle that enables me to honour them harmoniously. I am able to *live* each day, rather than just work. To me, nothing feels like work anymore.

I have always been someone who will work hard, earn my time off and have a great holiday or whatever it may be. I have now come to realise that that is a very old fashioned way of thinking. This is the 21st century, and times have changed. We have the ability to do what we want when we want and I intend to make the most of it.

As a business owner I have the key to open the door to whatever life I want for one very simple reason: I run my own diary! Up until now I had got it all completely wrong. With everything electronic, I found that I was filling all the white blanks in my diary with pointless work tasks that got me nowhere. I had to be doing something to do with work or I would feel guilty.

Now I work in bursts of high productivity. I see clients when I am on top form, write when I am in the mood and spend plenty time doing things I want to do. I create plenty of time in my day to devote to training and preparing good meals. I have my social life back and, despite wanting to improve it further by experiencing new things, it is definitely a marked improvement on the previous few years. And to top it all off, as a result of my new lifestyle, I make more money. The reason being that I took all the pressure off and started to value myself. When I did that, everything fell into place nicely.

My Story

I often hear the excuse "life gets in the way" for why so many people neglect their wellbeing. However, it is not life getting in the way. It is life *sailing away*. It is difficult to see at this stage of life because we are so wrapped up in ourselves that we are not realising what we are missing out on. Time flies by so quickly and before you know it, it has gone.

My reason for living is simple: I want to make the most of this short time we have here. I want to do so with great friends and experience great times. I want to be able to call people up each day to see what they fancy doing without being told they are "too busy". I want to create a community of fit and active entrepreneurs with the perfect work-life balance that they can enjoy every day. Most importantly though, I want to give something back.

TWO
What Is Success

> "Success is not the key to happiness. Happiness is the key to success. If you love what you are doing, you will be successful."
>
> **ALBERT SCHWEITZER**

Why do you want to be successful? Surprisingly, this is a question that only a small number of entrepreneurs can answer. I know why they want to be successful. The same reason that I wanted it so badly.

It was not all just about the money. It was what the money could do. Money can buy us whatever we want. Money can attempt to fill the void of insecurities we have in our lives. Driving around in a flash car can do a great job of papering over the cracks of our deeper issues but it is very often short-lived. It will never fix those issues. If anything, it will exacerbate them.

Having money can make it appear to others that we are a success. That we have made it in life. This does not make it feel loving though. Trying to impress other people is exhausting. We have become obsessed with wanting to be perceived as successful. I would not mind betting that in many cases out there, people would rather be *perceived* as a success than to actually *be* one. Probably because it is a lot easier to act flash than to build from the ground up.

I was so driven to become successful because I wanted to show the world what I could achieve. There were no high hopes for the pupils of the school I went to. It was as if the mantra was to move heaven and earth to get into a trade and do whatever you can to avoid prison. It was by no means the worst school in the world, but to say there were one or two unsavoury characters is an understatement.

Wanting to break the tradition of having a job, any job, and staying in it to retirement, I always believed there was more to life. That we can have and do so much. A sentiment that is unfortunately not shared by people whenever I go back to my home town. People think I am from another planet. They think I have lost the plot and cannot for the life of them understand why I will not settle for a life of mediocrity.

I also had to contend with growing up thinking I was academically inept. A few of my friends went to far better schools than I did. In fact I was the only one in my street of my age who went to a comprehensive school. This automatically installed me as the idiot among the group. I was secretly mocked by their pushy parents. It made me feel stupid so I unconsciously went along with it, not bothering to put any effort in at school because I did not see any point to it. Although putting no effort in for 13 years of schooling I still managed to achieve better than average grades.

The interesting thing is that deep down I always knew that the education system was not designed with me in mind. Teachers would state that you would need to get your head down and work hard so that you could leave school and get a good job. I felt like I was being de-valued by the system from such a young age.

This never sat right with me from the start. I was dead against authority and I just could not figure out why. However, at the same time I was far too afraid to speak up for fear of punishment. The system had me well and truly whipped. Eventually I did break though. Leading up to my GSCEs I flipped on one of my teachers right in the middle of class and absolutely fed it to him in front of everyone.

There was an abundance of pressure placed on us, and every school child for that matter, to get as good grades as possible. My perception at the time was that this was not for our sake, but theirs. The teachers. They had targets to hit. They did not care for us, they cared for their job security. That was how I felt and it further enhanced my disdain for authority.

Going into employment I carried this on. I have had several jobs and quite a lot of bosses. There were only two or three I had no conflict with, and those were the ones who treated me with respect and valued me as a person. The rest I viewed as idiots who wanted to exert the little bit of power they held to feed their ego.

I knew from early on in life that I could not be caged, and that I had my own ideas and my own ways of doing things. However, my home town community, the judgmental parents of supposedly smarter kids, selfish teachers and idiot bosses were the driving force behind me wanting to become successful. I wanted to show them what I could achieve and rub it in their faces.

It dawned on me that this just did not feel loving in any way. I was trying to be successful for the wrong reasons. To prove people wrong. As a result I was becoming such a show off. Look at me doing this, look at me doing that. Look at me, look at me. Look how amazing and wonderful my life is. Ego, ego, ego. All this did was build up frustration because all it was was fluff. All style and no substance.

In my observation of entrepreneurs over recent years, I believe that so many of them pursue success because of oppressive incidents or experiences in their lives. I wanted to make loads of money so that I could buy a life that all those people I mentioned previously could only dream of.

An observation I make in society is how we put celebrities on pedestals and are amazed by them. We are fascinated and obsessed with them. This is also true in the entrepreneurial world.

There are entrepreneurs and business owners out there who aspire to be the success story that is the flavour of the month. Follow this guru, listen to that leader, all of whom we hold in such high regard.

Adopting this attitude will only lead to frustration and hold you back. Yet I wanted these people to feel that way about me. Why aspire to be someone else when you are already you? Why consider yourself below others? Of course you can hold certain figures in high regard and learn from them, but they are just people. The same as you and me. No one is better or worse than you. Not believing that will only make you feel bad about yourself in one way or another.

As entrepreneurs we are together creating a fairer and more balanced society. More and more small businesses are cropping up everywhere now and corporations are beginning to lose their stranglehold on us. Yet so many entrepreneurs I meet have the mindset of these corporations and want, in some way, to rule the world.

It feels like we are stepping over one another to get what we all want. It does not matter who we hurt in the process, just so long as we are sorted. This contradicts the spirit of entrepreneurship in my view. I believe entrepreneurship is about solving problems, servicing humanity and creating a better world. It is about giving back.

As it stands, we are no different from anyone else in society. We are all so fixated with consumerism. We have to have everything. I am not knocking material wealth. I just believe that when that becomes our driving force, we distance ourselves from what success really is and what the important things in life are.

The world is changing and at such a fast pace. Everything is becoming more transparent and we are becoming wiser. Or more to the point, we are getting better at accessing our innate wisdom. I do believe that we are starting to find our way and tuning into our hearts a lot more.

One thing that prevents this is the idea of competition. As one of around 15,000 active Personal Trainers in the country, I am often asked what makes me different. We are *all* different: we all have our own way of doing things and there is no right or wrong answer in my industry, contrary to what many people may try to force upon you.

This is a message I put across when I teach trainers because they are given text books and expected to take everything in them as gospel. The first thing I tell them is to be sceptical of everything they learn. I tell them to make their own minds up and develop their own style of coaching and training. They will then attract the clients their methodology resonates with.

The first thing many entrepreneurs do is find out who their competition is then set out to beat them. The way I see it is that with seven billion people in the world, there is enough business to go around. However, competing with one another and trying to beat each other makes entrepreneurs feel successful.

That does not necessarily make one successful, though. Look what is sacrificed as a result. The care for the client, for a start, because it is not about them, it is about the glory. The fight with another human being. We emanate from a field of love so how can competing in business lead us to success? Competition, I believe, should be left in the realm of fitness – which I will explain in a later chapter.

Competing with other business owners for a slice of the pie is exhausting and completely unnecessary. Success does not need to be difficult. Success can be effortless if we only let go of the desire to feed our ego. When we look at the bigger picture and live by it, success will happen automatically. Chasing success, much like chasing money, is counter-productive.

Are we already successful? Yes, I believe we are. From a biological viewpoint we have beaten overwhelming odds to even be here. With so many millions of possible genetic combinations, it is you who won the race. Why overlook the amazing gift of life you already have? Understand that this is a success in itself.

For so long, success has been perceived to be the accumulation of material wealth, but that is only for other people's benefit, so they can be impressed by you. Success is not about impressing other people. Success is about how you feel about yourself. Success is about how much you give back.

In the current world of short-term gain, we are destroying the planet at an alarming rate. We are distancing ourselves from one another and alienating ourselves from our very essence of being. What so many fail to realise is that we are still reproducing despite this. What will be left for our grandchildren? And their grandchildren? And so on. How can we honestly deem ourselves to be successful if we are only in it for ourselves?

If we continue to live by the one-dimensional definition of success that is only about financial accumulation and short-term gain then it will only create a vicious circle. There is only so much we can buy. It will give us satisfaction that will only be short lived. Therefore we chase it more and more but the pleasure fades each time.

I believe that the time has now come for us to change the definition of success once and for all. It is high time we looked ourselves in the mirror and said that success is all about fulfilment and happiness. Being happy will breed success. Yet success will not necessarily breed happiness. In many cases, success can actually inhibit or even destroy happiness.

I shut myself off completely from the life I wanted to live. All in pursuit of so-called success. It left me unhappier than I was when I had even less. Sometimes we just have to look at these situations we find ourselves in and ask what on earth is the point? Why shut off our happiness completely just to earn the riches? The best things in life cannot be bought.

Over the coming chapters, I will share with you what I believe to be five key pillars that, when mastered, can help create a life that you really want to live. Big statement – but I do not meet very many happy people out there.

This process is for you and about you. However, it will also benefit others. By excelling at these steps and creating the happiest life possible, you will inspire more people to discover their own happiness. This is worth its weight in gold.

By honouring yourself and living the life that you want to live, you will bring into your world the right people. You will share your insights with others. You will be giving back and you will be creating a domino effect in so many lives. Another bold statement, but the world needs more love and happiness. The world needs us to come together and be one. It does not need more separation.

Now is the time to put everything into perspective and look at the bigger picture. A time to invest in yourself for the good of others. A time to be who you truly are and to live in your greatness. One day you will be able to look back and know that you did your bit to save humanity from self-destruction.

THREE
Step One - Meaning

"Human seeks to find meaning and feel frustration or vacuum if this desire remains unfulfilled."

VIKTOR FRANKL

You will find that a lot of Personal Trainers are starting to delve more into **mindset**. Psychology is a new beast for my peers and getting to grips with it is extremely important. I found myself going down the same route and became very interested in how the mind works. Personal development has been a love of mine since I got into the health and fitness industry.

When I first started out, I found that I was struggling with sales. I never expected for one second that I would have to sell. I thought I would just turn up to the gym on my first day and there would be a queue of people waiting there for Personal Training. If only it were that easy!

My friend, Jake, alerted me to the works of Brian Tracy and I was instantly hooked. I loved what he was saying and started believing more in myself. A new passion was uncovered and my confidence grew. I was reading books, watching YouTube clips and could sense how I was improving.

It was still a huge struggle for me, though. I just felt too conscious of looking stupid if I tried to sell during a consultation. Or I just could not bear any rejection – something I have since realised a lot of people struggle with. It became very frustrating; I spent so much time walking around the gym attempting to talk to people, but I just never could. I felt paralysed.

During a session with a client, a very successful salesman, I brought up the difficulty I had with sales. It just did not feel right and I guess deep down I did not believe I could provide value for their money. He gave me some excellent advice and even gave me his copy of *Psycho-Cybernetics* by Maxwell Maltz. It is one of my favourite books on the mind.

From here, my confidence grew again. I was able to become more assertive and stamp my authority on my clients. I charged for cancellations and I helped them get much better results. I had been far too soft and let clients walk all over me. Once I stepped up my game, they fell into line and soon started to adhere to my methodology.

At this point, I was oozing confidence; I admit that I fell into the trap of arrogance that is common among Personal Trainers. A lot of the time I thought I knew everything. I nipped that in the bud when I started to surround myself with more successful trainers and coaches. I was, though, building Personal Training businesses in double quick time.

I have worked at a few gyms in my time as a Personal Trainer and am not ashamed to admit I failed in a few of them. At the time I felt I did not really have what it took to succeed and ended up quitting. I became more successful when I became involved in personal development.

There was something of a Last Chance Saloon when I got a job at one gym. I had been offered a job in recruitment and turned it down to give Personal Training one last crack. I went in all guns blazing and built a sustainable business in under 12 weeks. In fact, I was the first trainer that club had ever had to hit over 100 sessions in a month. This felt good and certainly told me that I could do anything I wanted if I set my mind to it.

The next step for me was to have another go at Central London. Having previously flopped before, I wanted to prove to myself I could cut it in a tougher demographic. I also wanted to charge more! I transferred to a gym in Covent Garden and built a sustainable business in under nine weeks this time. I had the bit between my teeth and would stop at nothing to ensure I got it.

It was not all plain sailing but I got there. The trouble was it just was not enough for me. Call me ungrateful, but I wanted to make more money and have more of a social life. Working there gave me neither. It was incredibly frustrating and got me really down a lot of the time.

I started to take on more work teaching the Personal Training certification; this, combined with clients, meant I was making a lot more money than before. Yet I had even less of a social life than before. I did what I set out to do and I proved so many things to myself, but it did not take me long to realise that this just was not enough and that I had a calling I needed to honour. Out of desperation I hired an Elite Life Coach by the name of Tony J Selimi to help me uncover what my calling was and to help me build it. In all honesty I went for it on a bit of a whim because I thought it would distract me from the pit I had found myself in.

What I did not expect for one second, though, was just how much it would blow my mind. I was instantly re-energised and from the initial consultation started to get my spark back. I could not believe just how much clarity I would get almost immediately or how I could actually visualise in great detail what I wanted out of life.

I thought that coaching would take me to the next level. What it did was fast track me to the rooftop. I am not talking financially here. Of course my earnings have risen since, but I am referring to an all round improvement in all key areas of my life.

This is because Tony taught so much more than just about the mind. He taught me how to look deeper within myself; to help me discover true meaning in what I am about; what it is that I want and how I am going to get it..

This comes downs to values. What is it that I truly value in this world and how can I honour this? This is how you become successful. This is how you discover inner peace and true happiness. Honouring your own values instead of somebody else's. We are so very often bombarded with somebody else's agenda.

Once you discover what it is that you truly value in your world, everything falls into place nicely. The universe conspires to make everything happen for you. It really is as simple as that. By putting yourself first and honouring what is important to you, you can have whatever life you wish.

Of course, you have done the first part in electing a life that you are in control of by working for yourself. With this, however, it is very easy and even addictive to be continuously working. You have other parts of your world that you need to honour as well.

Let's say, for example, that one of your top values is your family. For many people it is at the very top. What do you do on a daily basis to honour that? Apart from merely bringing home the bacon? How much time do you spend each day playing with your kids? How much quality time do you spend with your spouse, on a daily basis?

Many of you reading this may look at it and say "Miller, you mad man! I am running a business in order to provide for my family!" Fine. Is it enough, though? Do you think the next generations need better nurturing these days? Especially when the world needs more love in a time of unprecedented change.

You are reading this book because health is important to you. You grew up with fitness levels through the roof and boundless energy. Running a business has wiped a lot of that away and you want to reclaim it. Therefore, how well are you honouring your health if you work all the hours under the sun so that you can provide for your family?

Would it not make a lot more sense to pull out all the stops to ensure that you minimise the risks of anything ever happening to you? For your family's sake? Since when was it ok to neglect a major cog in the machine that is your family's livelihood? You are part of your family as well, you know! A very big part.

I am putting it to you in this way for your own good. It really is not worth missing out on the best parts of your life just for the sake of working 24/7. Sure I could sit here and write about work/life balance, but without understanding what it is that you truly want from life it would just be a complete waste of time.

We need to start from within. Get to the core of our being and understand our purpose. From here it is about honouring that. Every. Single. Day.

Your values can, and most likely will, change over time. This is totally fine. Therefore keep revisiting your values and change what you feel is necessary. You will know if they are right based on how you feel. If there is ever a time when I feel frustrated or angry, I know it is because something is out of alignment somewhere.

In this case, all I need to do is journey back and see what I was doing or what I was not doing and then ask myself what I can do to change this going forward. For example, my time is valuable. I get angry with myself when I let my day sail by, and it does not feel very loving to be in this situation. Therefore, the next day I ensure that I have an action plan of what I want to achieve.

By improving my organisational skills and setting myself deadlines to complete work, I feel a lot better about things. It means I have completely removed that feeling of guilt when I step away from work for the day to enjoy some quality '*Me*' time.

Another time I lack productivity and let time sail by is when I have a few days off exercise. This is something I will be covering in the next chapter. There was a time recently when I suffered a bad tackle at football and had to lay off exercise for a few days to rest my ankle. I got virtually no work done in three days.

I could not honour my core value of health as well as I wanted to, therefore I could not honour my value of time as I would so wish. This made me feel quite low and frustrated. To add to the mix, when I exercise less, I do not eat as well as I usually would. It becomes a vicious circle!

Living by your values will cause controversy because we can be perceived as selfish. Putting yourself first is deemed as selfish. For some reason, we have people around us that will insist on us subordinating to their values. Then complain when we do not comply. Yet if we share different values then it will not feel loving on either side unless they are being communicated appropriately.

Talking of controversy, I made a statement recently that many people wanted to jump on. I stated that I believe that weight gain, illness and disease are the result of a lack of self worth. People can agree or disagree with that. It is what I believe to be true.

When we de-value ourselves and do not treat ourselves with the utmost respect and love, we open up a gateway of risks. We run the risk of getting ill. We bring the wrong people into our world and they drag us down. When we live in congruence with our values, we just emit love all around.

I recently interviewed Peter, a small business owner I met at an event. Peter is someone who honours his values at all times. He told me that every evening without fail, he goes for a walk with his family. Family being his highest value, he ensures that he spends quality time with his wife and children each and every day.

The significant thing about his approach is that they are out of the house, talking and communicating and, of course, getting some exercise. This is a huge difference to sitting in front of the television together night after night.

The added benefits to this is that he gets to unwind from his work and set himself up for the following day with a clearer mind. Not only that, but as he is committed to family time he has to ensure that his productivity levels are up to scratch so that his workload does not pile up. By honouring his highest value, Peter has improved the efficiency in the way he works.

Hopefully by now you are starting to build a picture in your mind of how important it is to value yourself fully. Love yourself fully. You are the player in the game they call life. Ensure that you treat yourself with the utmost respect. This will inspire those around you to fulfil their own greatness. It will breed love and respect for you from others.

Would you not just love to leave this world knowing you played a big part in helping others succeed and lead a fulfilling life? Would you not love to leave a legacy that showed the world what an incredible life you lived? Think about it.

FOUR
Step Two – Movement

"Motion is life."
HIPPOCRATES

As entrepreneurs, leading an active lifestyle can very easily be the least of our priorities. I know this myself as I skipped many a training session because I either had far too much work on or I was just too drained to be bothered to do anything. Sure, being on my feet all day was activity, but not as I would have wished. Certainly not the only activity needed for my goals.

However, I managed to overcome this by making some changes in my approach to exercise. As a result I was able to get myself back to those good old days of fitness that I had experienced before running a business. I decided that I would need to incorporate four key elements if I were to bring the glory days back. These four elements are, in my experience, the best way to achieve true fitness again.

Many entrepreneurs I speak to will reference bite-sized workouts that they can do from home. I am not suggesting spending hours doing exercise, I am just suggesting by showing exercise, and in essence, your body, a little more respect, you can really maximise your gains.

Variety

Having worked with over 200 clients in my time as a Personal Trainer, I have dealt with my fair share of common injuries. Everything from back pain to rehabilitation of an injury. In fact almost everyone I have worked with has had some kind of issue somewhere. Not only that, but things are getting much, much worse out there.

I love having variety in my own training and also that of my clients. It helps keep things fresh and it gives the body a chance to master a particular discipline then have appropriate rest from it. Growing up, I had always been something of an all-rounder. Though football is my main sport, I was also very good at distance running along with racket sports.

Since entering the fitness industry I have been getting involved with strength training and now practise Calisthenics from time to time. That variety not only keeps things interesting but also helps prevent and even fix certain injuries.

Over the years, I have taken a complete battering from football. I have had more injuries than hot dinners. I love spiriting and have always been lightning quick, but sometimes not quick enough and

Step Two – Movement

have felt the brunt of many a harsh challenge. I have suffered a shattered wrist, a hernia and had the bone in my big toe pointing in another direction. I have even torn the tissues around a disc in my lower back.

It has never deterred me, though. Being physically fit and active is something that I will never give up without a fight. No matter what age I get to. I have no intention of stopping. This, I believe, is the attitude required to help rid oneself of pain symptoms.

In this day and age, we have gotten far too soft. If something hurts we go crying away to our hiding place, wanting sympathy. I know this because it was always what I did. I wanted to come across as some kind of sporting hero. Injured in battle. The thing with that is, of course, soldiers are taught how to ignore pain and get on with it. I was just being a wimp.

I found that I had a very high success rate in helping my clients become pain free. The reason for this is that they started to move a lot more. This enables the brain to get feedback from the body to say that moving is safe and the perceived risk is not as high as first feared.

If you have ever found that you have had some kind of physical issue, let's say low back pain for example, it is very easy to stop any movement possible in order to "protect" the area. I know what that is like because that is exactly what I did when I had my back problem. However, minimising movement can very likely make things worse.

In simple terms, the less we move, the more our brains will start to 'erode' our overall ability to move. Therefore, what were minimal movements before, now become bigger movements that we are less able to handle, thus increasing the risk of further injury. Simple things like bending down or running for a bus become risky. Is that something you would have thought possible in your early 20s?

Movement is a huge factor in overcoming pain and musculoskeletal issues. However, I am not saying that you need to go dancing around immediately and to hell with pain. You may need to ease yourself in first. It could be that you need to spend some time on some mobility or flexibility work for example.

My client, Adam, a partner in a firm of solicitors, spent five years in the fitness wilderness and let his back pain take over. He loved playing racquet ball but knew that the condition he was in at the time would lead him to make matters worse. Not only that, but he refereed rugby most weekends. The first thing was to improve the mobility in his hips. This improvement in overall flexibility meant that he could move more efficiently, which recruited more muscle to assist with dynamic movement.

Over time, his aches and pains began to ease and he got himself into a racquet ball league at the health club. Now that he was training with me and also had a sport he enjoyed playing, he found that this leveraged his fitness levels and began refereeing rugby at a higher standard.

Enjoyment

Another client I worked with, David, came to see me to help him with his shoulder. Having suffered injury many years ago, he started to notice more and more issues with it whilst playing his favourite sport, volleyball. He stated that as he was "getting on a bit" he should probably just give it up.

I am quite against the idea of giving up something you love doing. Sure, we agreed that he would need some rest time away from the sport, but very often, giving something up can make the problem worse. We needed to improve the mobility of the shoulder joint whilst increasing the stability of his shoulder blade. Over time we were able to incorporate some pulling type exercises to increase his strength.

Had he have stopped playing for good, I have no doubt that he would have tried many other sports or physical activities to fill the void. This is great because it gives the body a chance to learn new movements and adapt to different disciplines. However, if the same enjoyment is not experienced then it could be easy to gradually fall out of the habit.

I am still a member of a gym despite the fact that I have a lot of variety in my training diary. I go to yoga classes and I do some heavy training as well. Strength training is something that I love doing, but I must admit that it can be difficult to motivate myself sometimes – though I will explain later the importance of it.

When I go to the gym for a heavy workout I tend to just stick to one main lift with maybe a couple of smaller exercises. In all honesty, I am just trying to get it over with as quickly as possible so that I can hit the sauna and steam room.

Despite the need to get it done quickly, I find that I have rest periods between sets that are far too long. I lack the motivation to lift whilst I am by myself. In fact, there have been times when I have reduced the number of sets and reps I had planned to do just so I could get the hell out of there!

As a Personal Trainer it can sometimes be difficult to avoid the ego of the best way to do this and that. Usually because some guru somewhere has said so. There is a lot of in-fighting in this industry in which people who enjoy certain disciplines will criticise those who enjoy something completely different.

What so very many people fail to realise is that people like what they like. As long as they are giving it their all, they are achieving the fitness that they want to achieve.

Step Two – Movement

I am always asked what the best type of exercise is. My reply is always the same. I tell people to do what they enjoy, because they will commit to it and be consistent. However, as I stated earlier, variety is important so I suggest picking two or three activities.

I have a love of sprinting. I could join a club and race people. It would certainly be very competitive. However, I do also love playing football. For me it is a win-win situation. And it also adds a little bit of variety too because football requires a lot of changing direction and applying so many different movement patterns.

When I train for strength I try to go with my friend and fellow Personal Trainer, James. He competes in strongman events and is completely addicted to this discipline. This makes me enjoy it even more because I can feed off of his energy and enthusiasm. Also, because he is twice my size I find myself having to push a lot harder than I would by myself just so I can save a bit of face.

I have rediscovered the joy of running, I have found myself bouldering very regularly and I love doing yoga. The point is that I have a range of sports and activities that I love doing and as a result they are all very important to me. I do not dread any of them; I love the feeling after each one and they take pride of place in my diary.

After leaving our younger years, many of us find ourselves using only the gym to stay fit. Gyms are great, but I see so many people stick to the same old machines and routines. I applaud the intention but now it is time to spice things up a little!

Strength

I believe that **strength** is one of the most overlooked components to true fitness. And for a number of reasons too. Firstly, fear. Lifting heavy weights has risks. Not performing with the correct technique can leave many people fearing it altogether. This is due to the possibility of injury or having previously been injured training in a similar way.

I have recently been working with a guy who spent a long time bed-ridden as a result of loading up too much weight for a back squat and deadlift. He was told that he would need surgery to repair the damage to his spine, but was heavily against the idea and felt that a more natural form of rehabilitation would be more appropriate.

We eased him in to a graded exposure of movement patterns before starting to work on exercise technique without any resistance. We made sure that he could stand with good posture and move in optimal alignment. We have since been looking at the psychological aspect whereby he has developed a fear of movement as a result of the injury.

When we experience pain we tend to store this experience and create habits and behaviours that try to protect us from

Step Two – Movement

experiencing this pain again. Therefore it is important to build confidence back into movement gradually in order for the brain to accept that the risk is not quite as bad as initially feared.

Another reason that strength training is overlooked is because it can be incredibly challenging. Forgive me for saying so, but I believe that we have become lazier in this day and age, as well as soft. It is far easier to go for a run or jump on a cardio machine in the gym and claim to be fit.

Lastly, I have had potential clients who claim that they do not want to bulk up. Strength training does not necessarily have to spark that response in the body. I can deadlift twice my own body weight, but am stick thin. Packing on serious lean muscle mass will involve eating serious amounts of food.

There appears to be a misunderstanding around resistance training. There is a difference between body-building and strength training. Sure, it all involves lifting weights but bodybuilding is a serious competitive sport. It involves high volume and isolating certain muscles to focus on increasing their size. Strength training is about going heavy for low reps on what are known as compound exercises whereby two or more joints are moving which uses several muscles at the same time.

Of all the reasons as to why strength training is overlooked, I believe the biggest is the fact that the benefits are not understood well enough. External benefits involve having a lean physique with a low percentage of body fat; a strong heart function; better performance in your favourite sports and activities; more power.

For me though, it is the feeling of *being* strong. How it affects us internally. Being strong makes us feel great inside. And that radiates outward. It gives us an inner belief and greater confidence. It shows others around you that you care about yourself, that you love yourself. Fit body, fit mind. Strong body, strong mind.

Being strong means you mean business. You own the room when you go into meetings. You are the boss. Respecting yourself means that others will respect you. You will ooze confidence knowing that you possess sheer strength.

You will also find that you have lowered the risk of injury too. Going through a range of different strength exercises will help to make you robust enough to handle what anything else can throw at you. You will be fearless in your pursuit of all round success.

Not only can strength training decrease injury risk, it can also help you overcome existing pain. Take my client Scott, for example. In his early 20s, Scott was very much into his combat sports as well as heavy lifting in the gym. Fast forward 15 years and the little issues that flared up back then were now beginning to surface all too regularly. Knee pain, shoulder pain and lower back pain.

Scott runs his own brokerage firm and knew he needed to improve his energy levels, so he got himself back to the gym. As a result of these issues, he was very cautious about what he did and only really went through the motions with his training. He approached me to help him overcome all this and get back some of that power from days gone by.

We worked a lot on improving his movement as well as exercise technique, and started to build the foundations of strength. Within next to no time he realised that all those issues had disappeared, which meant he could really start excelling. It took a while but we got him deadlifting two and a half times his own bodyweight for three reps. He felt like a powerhouse again.

Competition

Throughout my school days I used to kill it in P E. Not to brag, but I was pretty darn good at everything. That is because I had to be. I had people breathing down my neck and there is no way I would be beaten. I was far too competitive. I had to win everything.

To this day I am still very good friends with my biggest fitness rival, Ben. We have mellowed these days, and given that we play in the same football team we do not have a great deal to compete over now. However, during school, it was me versus him.

When it came to cross-country running we always made a pact with each other to run together and wipe the others out of the water. We found that the last few hundred yards was a flat out race. I am pretty sure I won all of them; at least, that is how I like to remember it!

Upon turning 16, we joined the gym and got to use all those fancy machines. We always found ourselves on the rower at the same time and somehow setting up the same distance. A casual start followed by greater intensity. Checking each other's pace out of our periphery. I won those races too!

Out on our bikes it was down to who could ride up the hill in the highest gear. Not only that, but who could actually get up it first. He may have had the edge on me in that one. Of course I let him win!

What I realised is that we both did each other a huge favour. By being so competitive with one another, our fitness levels were far better than anyone else's in our year – probably even the school, because neither of us smoked or drank back then.

I firmly believe that being so competitive has kept me very fit, not to mention slim. Even throughout the inconsistency of my training, I would claw it back in next to no time at all. Also, I spent the years aged 16-25 going out drinking all the time. I believe that I have offset some of the damage as a result of my younger years.

As we get a bit older, we tend not to be as competitive. I know I have certainly chilled out more. However, I had noticed that I was starting to slip. I decided to get back into football again because it was the perfect way for me to keep doing my sprints.

Step Two – Movement

Of course I could go to the park to sprint or even join an athletics club, as I mentioned, but I get a great deal of satisfaction tearing past the opposition right back. Ryan Giggs, eat your heart out! Knowing I have someone chasing me who wants to break my legs really helps keep me on my toes. Excuse the pun.

Simon, a partner in a business analytics firm, is one of my older clients. Approaching 50, Simon values his health and fitness very much. In fact, he always has. This attitude has served him very well as he came to me wanting to train for climbing Denali in Alaska.

This is not competition, but it is certainly an event that requires the absolute best from an individual. A gruelling 10-day climb to the summit in freezing conditions, it requires a great deal of focus and has very little margin for error. Simon needed to train for this as if it was competitive, or who knows what could happen.

It is time for you to reignite that fire within that wants to beat everyone in sight and achieve incredible feats of fitness. That feeling of winning. That fear of losing. Then you will start to notice the simple things becoming so much easier. You will notice just how much your confidence increases in all areas of your life.

FIVE

Step Three – Mindful Meals

"The food you eat can either be the safest and most powerful form of medicine, or the slowest form of poison."

ANN WIGMORE

These days you cannot move for health products. They are everywhere and shoved down your throat, in more ways than one. This would be acceptable were it not for the shameless pursuit of money that a lot of companies apply.

It is very easy for them to give us all these stories about how their products benefit us. It is also very easy for us to fall for it. We buy all these products and feel no better off as a result. Sure, there are some improvements but in a lot of people they are very short lived.

I am referring to products that you might find in health food shops that are supposedly 'essential' for us, but worse are the products you find in not so healthy shops that claim to be healthy, such as health bars that have gone through an abundance of processing. It is just all junk to me.

I am not quite sure why the idea of living a healthy lifestyle is no longer the norm. It is as if there are shortcuts to true health popping up everywhere. It is all just a ploy to take people's money with no intention to do good. Then we are being told that they are "passionate" about health and wellness and want to "help" people.

As a Personal Trainer, I have so many people try to sell me on to their multi-level marketing programmes. A few years back I decided to go ahead with one of them and I was excited. Among all of them out there, this was the only one that appeared to hold any credibility.

I was using the products regularly and felt great. Certainly better than I had been feeling as a result of early mornings and long days. I cannot deny that the extra boost of vitamins helped me throughout my day.

However, one day, I looked at the ingredients of some of the products and saw words that I could not pronounce. What I also discovered was that I was not all that bothered if my diet slipped a bit at times because I had these supplements to back me up.

That is exactly the way they want us to think. They will cite the reduction in the quality of our food over the last century to ensure we keep buying their products. It is a one billion pound industry because it has been marketed extremely well.

The knock-on effect is that we continue to let our diets slip. We adopt this idea that we can continue to eat meat that has been heavily injected with antibiotics and steroids. To continue to eat foods containing vast amounts of sugar.

I gave these vitamins up, and also the business that went alongside it. I just focused more on eating as well as I could. I made sure I got what I needed from high quality foods. No surprises for guessing that I feel even better as a result.

Business Man

As someone who runs a business, I am adamant that I need to fuel my body with the right foods. Sure I have the occasional blow out; I am only human. However, I understand the necessity of ensuring that my body is well equipped to handle what business ownership throws at me.

Productivity is key when it comes to running a business. We need to ensure that we squeeze as much as we possibly can out of every situation. For this, energy levels are incredibly important. Living off sandwiches for lunch, sugar for breakfast and wine for dinner is not going to serve us well in the long run.

It is all too easy to cite business lunches and networking events as an excuse to indulge. In my humble opinion, if that is due to pressure thrust upon you by prospect or client meetings, then they are not the type of client that you want. It will only lead to the detriment of your business.

If you are genuinely serious about your business and about achieving all round success in your life then these are the people you do not want around you. Regardless of how big their cheque book is. How can you deliver on your promises to that client, and other clients for that matter, if you slow yourself down through poor nutrition?

This is something I experienced whilst working long hours. I was fuelling myself with chocolate bars and cookies in between meals to make up for my lack of sleep. I had to get really clever about hiding yawns in front of clients. Not only that but it was just plainly obvious at times that I did not want to be there.

Feeling like this was horrible. It did not feel very loving to myself or to my client. I just could not give my absolute best and the service I wanted to. Not only that but it would affect my sleep. I am a very deep sleeper, but coupled with feasting on junk right up until late I felt like I had been beaten up every morning when I woke.

It soon became obvious that I was reaching for all the junk food as a result of the long working hours. I will be covering stress and social interaction in later chapters but it was the overwhelm of the former and the disappearance of the latter that got me reaching for the sugar. Not to mention the inconsistency with my own fitness training.

Chocolate was definitely my vice. That and Krispy Kreme doughnuts. I could demolish a dozen of those in no time at all. I would use going out for a meal or to the cinema as an excuse to go mad with food. I would justify to myself that it was OK because I was out.

What I found was that I would carry on this idea throughout the weekend and then set an intention to start again Monday. Come Monday evening I would have a couple of chocolate bars which became a habit throughout the week. Before I knew it, it was Friday night again and time to binge.

All this did was make me feel sluggish and tired. My energy levels wavered so much that I just could not function how I wished. I felt that food had a real hold over me which was something I could never beat. As soon as I thought of something sugary, my mind would keep teasing me until I caved in.

Being pretty slim throughout my whole life, I have not only been able to get away with eating junk up to my late 20s but it also meant I could hide it from people. I was dishing out advice and holding clients accountable, but I was a complete hypocrite. Telling clients to cut back on certain things knowing full well that after that session I was going to buy a pack of Oreos. Not the example you would wish from your Personal Trainer.

Aesthetics are important to me, but I see them as an added bonus to being physically fit and eating well. Of course I want to look good and will always want to have a visible six pack at any age. I will never fall into the trap of the dreaded beer gut. Therefore I knew I needed to conquer my issue with food.

I have always been health conscious but it has only been since I got into the health and fitness industry that I actually started to know anything about nutrition. I always fell for all the rubbish that is out there when it comes to advertising so-called health products.

During sixth form, I worked at McDonalds; due to the never ending food fights and providing the source of income for my boozy nights out, it was by far the best job I have ever had. The trouble is that the food is incredibly addictive. We were allowed one meal every shift but we certainly abused that rule!

I have not eaten the stuff for quite some time now, but I do believe that having spent so long immersed in it is part of the reason for my binge eating. I made several efforts to not eat the stuff, including going across to the petrol station next door every day to buy a sandwich and a packet of crisps. To me that was the healthier option.

My coworkers would mock my attempts to be 'healthy' so it was not long until I succumbed to burgers and fries again. And chicken nuggets. And milkshakes. And ice cream. You get the picture. No matter what stage of life we are at, though, there are plenty of people out there who want to derail our good intentions.

Value Thyself

This is where **values** come back to the fore. When we look at honouring our values it means we are honouring ourselves. This means that we love ourselves and ensure that we treat our bodies with the utmost love. By acting in this way we are able to experience true health.

Starting out as a Personal Trainer I was very soft on clients. They would give me their excuses and I would empathise. This is because I had been in that position myself and understood where they were coming from. It did not take too long to figure out that this attitude was only to the detriment of my clients and also myself.

I began toughening up – but knew I had to start with myself. I was determined to stay strong and fight my food demons. This goes way beyond willpower, though. This is about heart and knowing that in order to succeed in all key areas of my life I needed to love myself so much more.

A huge turning point for me was deciding to order the healthiest thing on the menu whenever I was out. My social life was not exactly that of some A-list celebrity but I would have meals out and go to networking events or workshops, so plenty of times when I could have been excused for eating whatever I wanted.

One big factor with this approach was the fact that I became less greedy. People often think I have hollow legs due to the amount I can eat. However, it really is nothing more than just plain greed. Choosing the healthiest thing on the menu was something I had accepted and knew it was the best thing to do for my own good.

This soon became a habit, and barring the odd time when I know I will not be racked with guilt, I would say that virtually every meal I have is the healthiest option. Of course, depending on where I go it would be very easy to question just how healthy something actually is, but knowing that I am sticking to my intention gives me greater peace of mind.

My client Robin, who owns a company that develops business strategies for entrepreneurs, found that he had put a lot of weight on since becoming a father for the first time. He still needs to keep up appearances at networking events and client meetings, so I suggested this little tip. He shifted a stone in under two months and has kept it off.

One of my huge successes with clients is to get them to complete a seven-day food diary upon starting my coaching programme. This is the first stage of nutrition and is extremely effective. It often shows up some very interesting results.

A food diary filled out in the initial stages of coaching tells me an awful lot about a client. It will go one of two ways: either I am left

Step Three – Mindful Meals

chasing the client for it, which then involves a serious chat. Or it highlights to the client just exactly what they do eat.

I encouraged two of my friends from my football team to fill out a food diary. I was curious to see what the outcome would be. The first one had a great success in being completely honest, having a stark realisation and beginning to make changes in his life. He lost over a stone in under two months. It was not quite as successful for the other chap. Having written out what can only be described as the entire contents of a vending machine on day one, he soon gave up.

When I tasked my client Tim, another broker, with filling in a food diary, it raised his awareness on what he was actually consuming. So much so that he started to lose weight before I even gave him his first action step. With his new found awareness he was able to cut out some of the bad foods he had been eating and felt immediate benefits. With a little bit of fine tuning on my part, he ended up losing three stone in less than six months.

Is That All

If only it was as simple as picking the healthiest meal when out dining and keeping a food diary. Well eventually it is, although there is still a lot to cover and nutrition goes a lot deeper. As business owners, we deal with a fair amount of stress and a lack of time –

the subjects of the next chapter. These can have a dramatic effect on our food choices. More than you would think.

One more spanner to throw in the works is tiredness. When I am tired, I start reaching for the sugars and the comfort foods. Anything to pick me up and give me an instant hit. Of course this is counter-productive because it hits me hard a little later. It can end up being a vicious circle and lead you to write the whole day off completely. All these vicious circles; it is no wonder we almost spiral out of control.

There are three key drivers behind eating.

First, we are **hungry**. It has been a while and the stomach starts to rumble. Off we go to get some food.

The second is that our body needs **nutrients**. Given the choices of food these days, it is often difficult to take in what we actually require.

The third driver is **emotional**. This is a very big deal indeed and one that we shall be covering in depth.

What I started to do with myself and then coach clients about is to get to the root of every food choice. This is often referred to as 'Mindful Eating'. It has made a huge difference to not only mine but to my clients' results too. It has become an extremely effective tool in my coaching practice.

Step Three – Mindful Meals

I do not believe for one second that there is a correct diet for us all to follow. For example, I gave up meat not so long ago and noticed my energy levels go through the roof. However, I am not suggesting that this should be the way for everybody. We are all different and require different things.

My view is that our bodies know what they need. We just need to improve that connection to our bodies' wisdom. External factors such as stress, tiredness and long hours will only result in that link becoming, let's say, inaccurate.

Mindful eating is about checking in with oneself to ascertain why we eat what we eat and what mood we were in before and after. If not addressed properly it can be a very slippery slope. I was able to figure this out in my early years of business ownership. You may have been living off the stresses and strains for several years and eating accordingly.

By knowing what exactly was the driver, we can go back and ensure we handle it better the next time a similar situation arises. For example, if it was a stressful episode that led to eating something you perhaps should not have done, what exactly was that stressful moment? Is it likely to happen again? How can you better prepare for when it does? Can you prevent it from happening again?

Whatever the situation, the point is that nothing is worth risking your health over. This behaviour of eating out of consolation will only trap us further. This is how I felt when I just could not shake my need for sugar and other rubbish. It made me feel terrible afterwards.

In essence, food is fuel. Of course we are going to have holidays and weekends away where perhaps the bar is lowered to some degree. However, the point is that we need to be on top form all the other times. We need energy and lots of it. With greater energy we are in control.

How much more productive do you think you would be if you ate wholesome, nutritious foods and stayed well hydrated? You would have a clearer mind for sure and would be much more alert. What effect would this have on your business?

SIX

Step Four – Managing (Time and Stress)

"Organisation isn't about perfection; it's about efficiency, reducing stress and clutter, saving time and money and improving your overall quality of life."

CHRISTINA SCALISE

Running a business means that we have to manage ourselves well. With greater internal organisation we are able to create better external results. There are so many minor factors that need taking care of when it comes to business ownership but there are also a couple of very big and important aspects that need to be dealt with first.

I am, of course, referring to the management of time and the management of stress. I have paired these two because I believe that they go hand in hand. Also, for me, they are the two most important parts of running a business.

Time

A recent survey I conducted of over 1,000 entrepreneurs highlighted that a lack of time was the biggest factor when it came to keeping fit and healthy whilst running a business.

I was no different. I would find any excuse I could to justify missing training sessions for example. There was always something I needed to do for the business. Whether it be tweaking my website or having to respond to emails. I look back now and think of all the time I wasted just messing about with low-value tasks that really would hardly have made a difference.

In all honesty, I think the biggest reason for me was that I never really wanted to train alone. Therefore I had no motivation. I also feel that perhaps I had always taken my fitness for granted and just expected it to remain. Therefore it would not matter too much if I missed sessions because I knew I could get sharp again in next to no time.

There is no doubt that we will always free up time, and money, for what we value. With exercise and eating well, it is very difficult to notice the immediate value. Whereas booking in a client meeting can potentially yield greater value from that time. What you will find with that, however, is that over time, we may increase our profits but we will have nothing to spend it on other than private doctors, physiotherapists or nutritional therapists, to name but a few.

Step Four – Managing (Time and Stress)

What I have managed to discover very early in my life and career is that there is no end goal in life. It is not like a computer game that you can get past all the levels of and complete the whole thing. Life is a journey. It gets much, much harder the longer we go on if we keep neglecting the most important thing. Ourself.

You do not need me to tell you about how many people out there on their deathbeds wished they had lived more and got more out of life. Bearing in mind we are talking about previous generations from a whole other era. Times are different now. We have found ourselves caught up in consumerism and competition with our fellow man.

The knock on effect is that we have to work ourselves into the ground for one of two reasons. The first is **survival**. As entrepreneurs we are different from the rest of the working society. It is a hard trend to buck but the fact remains that we do find ourselves in survival mode very often. The second reason is that we are trying to accumulate as many riches as possible.

That is what I wanted. I wanted the flash cars and big money so that I could show off. Look at me, look at what I made of myself. Truth be told, constantly thinking this way never really made me feel good about myself. I was too caught up in wanting to impress people and wanting success so badly. As soon as I let go of the fear of judgement I started to enjoy life a lot more.

It really is quite incredible that these days, with the amount of access we have to anywhere in the world and the key to experience whatever we want, we still get bogged down in this competitive mindset. Therefore our time gets taken up by so many things that will get us nowhere. And we sit around scratching our heads wondering how life sailed by so fast.

Money comes and goes. We can make as much or as little of it as we wish. Time is what we will never get back. I was always taking time for granted. I felt as if I had an unlimited amount of time and it would not matter if I devoted myself to my work for as long as it took to succeed. What we have to ask ourselves is, is it really worth it? What are we missing out on?

When we are not working, we feel guilty. You are responsible for your own livelihood and in many cases for that of your family too. We have surrendered to our mission and we need to ensure we pull through and make it work. However, is it really necessary to be checking emails constantly? Is it really fair to have work on our minds when we are with family and friends?

How much time do you give to the things in life that are of equal or even greater importance to your work? What message does it send to your children if you are working all the hours under the sun? What are you telling yourself if you just sit idly by and let your life sail past you in double quick time?

Step Four – Managing (Time and Stress)

My dad is a teacher and I remember him coming home after seven o'clock every evening and marking books until 10pm. Then again at the weekends, toiling away. I grew up thinking that working life is hard and that if you want to get anywhere in life, you need to put the effort in and clock up the hours.

It took me 29 years to realise that that is flawed logic. Working hard does not work. It is a dated model that is no longer suited to where we are now in the 21st century. It is also a model that is most definitely not suited to the wonderful world of entrepreneurship.

The way I see it is that working long hours will soon become a thing of the past. We are coming to a point in time now where *time* is the new *money*. We are beginning to value every precious moment we have on this planet because we are not here for very long, coupled with the fact that we cannot take anything with us.

I believe that the way we spend our time says so much about us. I immersed myself in my own work and did virtually nothing for the first three years of my new career in health and fitness. The fact was, however, I was hiding from something. I was so determined to become successful and looking back now that was because I was insecure with whom I actually was. It led to a fair amount of stress.

It felt as if there was something I needed to prove to the world. It was as if I wanted everyone to look at me and be impressed. Truth be told, I am not impressed with those who flaunt their wealth. It is a real off-put. I am impressed beyond measure with those who have all-round success and are gracious and humble with it.

The key was in being authentic to my true self. Deep down I am not a flash person, nor do I have a desire to show off. Growing up, I had always acted that way for popularity. Now I am realising that I care more for the wellbeing of humanity. I am dedicated and driven to create all-round success in my life so that I can help, teach and inspire others to create it in theirs. The riches along the way become just a bonus rather than the driving force.

Now my time is spent accordingly. I give equal worth, effort and time into growing myself as well as my business aspirations. In essence, the two go hand in hand. Being driven in this way means that I spend very little time doing what most of society does. For example watching television. Of course there are one or two shows I love watching and very occasionally I will watch them if I want to just chill out.

The point is that we do find ourselves wasting an awful lot of time doing things that create no value in our lives. Do we really need to spend time watching the latest series of a popular programme or could we be writing a book? Could we prepare our food for the next day? Could we exercise?

The idea that there is no time to fit everything in that we want to is just plain rubbish. It is no more than a poor excuse for letting oneself go. As I mentioned earlier, we will always make time for what we value. Therefore it is time to take stock of what we genuinely value in this world and start honouring those values.

I am determined to fulfil my potential. I am on a mission of self-mastery. This is because I believe that our spirit comes back and I want to give mine a head start in the next life. All so that I can continue to fulfil my long-term vision. We came here to learn and to grow, not to let life whizz by in a heartbeat.

I want to live to be 100 years old. That really is not a long time at all on Planet Earth. Most will live to their 70s and 80s and as the way things are going it will be in poor health. Would it not mean so much to you to make the most of your time here and maximise every second you have?

Stress

My friend Rob told me the story of how his father had worked so hard for his entire career in order to give his children the best possible start in life. They had a great education and everything they could possibly wish for. Rob's father passed away just six months after retiring. Rob tells me that he would have given up all the luxuries in his upbringing to have spent another five years with his dad in retirement.

My own (biological) dad died when I was four years old. Having spent several years battling health issues, his body finally gave up on him. He was 47 when a fatal heart attack struck one night. That is no age at all.

Stress can show up in so many ways. For example, it can cloud our thinking, it can drain our energy and it can affect our moods. All things I have gone through as a business owner, and I am sure you have too. We have all been there and quite frankly it does nothing but hold us back.

The pursuit of success really does make us go crazy sometimes. We deal with constant frustration and work ourselves up into a pit of anger. Lashing out at anyone we possibly can. We feel as though no one understands what we go through.

Of course, everything we go through is of our own doing. We create our own mess and curse the world when we feel as though it is not going our way. Yet what we fail to realise is that we signed up for it. We knew that entrepreneurship would be unpredictable. We knew it would not necessarily be easy.

I failed to see just how lucky I already was. I had everything I could wish for. A good income, my own diary and I could wear what I wanted to work. Yet it just was not enough for some reason. I kept chasing more and more, although I still had no idea what I really wanted. I would get so worked up with things that it just left me in a constant state of frustration and despair.

Step Four - Managing (Time and Stress)

Not having the clarity on how I actually wanted to live my life and what I wanted to get out of it would lead me to chasing greater riches. I observe this behaviour in so many entrepreneurs. It amazes me just how few entrepreneurs understand just how lucky they are. To have complete freedom of choice in our lives when the rest of society gets bossed around is surely enough to make us happy, right?

It took me quite some time to realise this. And while I was getting round to this, all it did was hold me back. Going around in circles and putting myself under unrelenting pressure to achieve something I was completely unclear about. I had no sense of direction. This is another behaviour I see in so many entrepreneurs. They have a great idea and the drive but fail to actually see where they want to take it.

In my case, it was a lack of belief in the value I could offer that really held me back. I just could not see how I could be successful as a Personal Trainer. In a massively devalued profession, I found myself getting dragged back with all the other trainers out there who do not believe in, or value, what they do.

Not having belief in myself was incredibly stressful. I would scour the internet for motivational gurus and get myself all built up and energised, only to find myself deflated when it came to taking action on something. I would get really worked up when it came to having to sell. I was not confident in my ability to sell, purely because I was not confident in the service I was offering.

When it came to keeping myself fit I would lose energy, strength and power. Therefore I would find myself deflated when I was not able to train the way I knew I could. Another reason I would skip sessions a lot of the time was the fear of under-performing. It was not a nice feeling at all, the reason for which I just could not figure out at the time.

Then there is **nutrition**. Despite all my best intentions to have healthy meals and ensure I got my full quota of nutritious foods in, I just could not stop the bingeing. Many people would try to justify this for me by saying that it did not matter too much as I ate healthily most of the time anyway. For me this was not good enough.

I just could not overcome my addiction for sugar. It was relentless. Every single day I would be scoffing chocolate bars and biscuits, to the point where I would get so full up yet still wanted more. It gave me a good hit but then made me feel dreadful very soon after. Of course, there are plenty worse things out there to be addicted to but like everything else, it would kill me slowly.

As a business owner though, **stress** can have the biggest effect on another extremely important aspect. Productivity. Tension blocks our creativity and will slow us down. This in turn will just hold us back. We are so fixated on becoming successful yet are going about it in completely the wrong way.

Step Four – Managing (Time and Stress)

With tension ever-increasing to the point of overflow, we find ourselves unable to think and act with a clear mind. Our decision-making takes a hit and this affects us in our business dealings. This in turn just makes us even more stressed. Another vicious circle to worry about. All the while our health becomes that little bit more affected.

We then become distant and have our heads elsewhere when we are in the company of our families or with our friends, not giving them our full attention or enjoying the present moment. Always with something on our minds. Unable to switch off. Is this really how you want to live your life? Is this even living at all? Is it really worth feeling like this?

My client Melanie who, despite running her business from home, always found herself in a state of stress. So much so that when she gets ill, it really hits her hard. Hardly surprising given that after a few days off she once returned to over 400 emails. I will discuss emails in a later chapter but I think that amount highly unnecessary.

Melanie's biggest stress reliever is exercise. Using her warm up time to tell me about the trials and tribulations of her work allows her to shift the worry that very often hangs over her. This sets her up nicely to get some good effective training in and leave the session feeling great and ready to tackle the workload.

We are extremely lucky and privileged to be living in the western world with so much opportunity right in front of us. Not only that, but sometimes we need to sit back and think, what really is the worst that can happen? We are never going to starve, we will always have a roof over our heads. We will always have the gift of life.

However, is it really losing everything that we fear the most? Or is it more the fear of not having everything? Sometimes we chase so much material wealth that we are completely blind to the destruction that we are creating for ourselves and those around us. Instead of stabilising what we already have and building it organically, we focus only on the bigger picture and ignore the most important things.

In my example, I was chasing so much success that I was spending money I did not even have. Granted, I was not going out and blowing it on cars and fancy champagne but I was going on courses, workshops and events that promised the earth. I was a sucker for the promise of success that all these coaching programmes claimed to offer.

There were good and bad ones, but ultimately it was not really worth the debt I accumulated in the process. It left me playing catch up in my business life and guess what, created even more stress for me. Not only did I need to start applying what I had learned from several different coaches but I was quite a few quid in the hole and seriously worried.

Step Four – Managing (Time and Stress)

I now understand that all of these programmes were designed with one thing in mind. To help entrepreneurs make more money. I am not knocking that. Money is important, of course it is. However, I question the intent of these coaches and it was quite evident that they just prey on the weak. Chasing money and having it as the driving force will only lead to frustration and lack.

Constantly believing that you need more money will only create the idea in your mind that you have **scarcity**. This is what you will attract as a result: even more scarcity. In my example, I was just throwing money around trying to make it rich. This set me back as it meant I needed to pay off debts. This is what I mean about being grateful for what we already have or we will end up creating destruction in our already amazing lives.

It meant I was not making the money I wanted for one very simple reason. I was not valuing money. I was treating it with a complete lack of respect and then just expecting more to come to me as a result. I was living in 'Cloud Cuckoo Land' with that attitude. All it did was compound my stress.

The best money I have ever spent was in hiring Tony as my coach. One of the first things he said to me was to let go of the need to make money. Take that pressure off from needing to pay bills and anything else. When you place a need onto something it will inhibit your pursuit of it. Once I got my head around this and changed my thought process, things started to look up for me financially.

SEVEN
Step Five – Madness

> "And in the end, it's not the years in your life that count. It's the life in your years."
> **ABRAHAM LINCOLN**

This is my favourite one of all. That is because this is all about fun. It is about living life to the full and enjoying each and every day. What is life if we cannot enjoy it? What is it that we really want to do in life? What stops us from living each day the way we want to? These are questions that I was asking of myself and also of so many entrepreneurs.

It is no surprise that on the whole the answers I was getting to this question were things like: financial independence, passive income, work/life balance. This led me to one very simple conclusion on what we all want from life. To live more. It really is as simple as that. To squeeze more out of this crazy thing called life.

Though I never really knew at the time why I busted a gut when I started my business and always wanted more, I look back now and realise why. Deep down I just wanted to *experience* more. I had been in Australia for so long that coming home felt like I needed to fall in with the rest of society and follow the standard path of marriage and mortgage. In all honesty though, being in my 20s I really could not think of anything worse.

All of my friends would question my motives, but I always see the bigger picture in life. Working nine to five would bore the life out of me, as would watching television all evening and drinking all weekend. I had gotten over that phase in Australia. Now I look around at so many people who are stuck in this rut, the only way of living they have ever known, which is now increasingly hard to escape from.

This is not a life that I envy, nor one that I could bear to live. However, for quite some time, I was not even doing a fraction of those things. In fact, a drunken night out or two would have been a welcome break in the monotony of working ridiculously long hours in the pursuit of what can only be described as a life of frustration, anger and despair.

While the rest of society went to work and had routine in their life, I had nothing but work. All the time thinking that I was the smart one for embarking on business ownership. How wrong I was at the time. For three years of my late 20s I did nothing but work, missing out on so many things. Yes, I had the odd holiday and such but in all honesty I was just letting time sail by and achieving nothing at all.

Step Five – Madness

Even if I wanted to go out at the weekend to get drunk I was too shattered to even bother. I would spend Saturdays and even a lot of Sundays working and any chance I got to sit down I would grab with both hands and just dumb my brain with mindless television. Embroiling myself in the complete and utter junk we have to suffer every time we grab the remote.

I have always loved playing football. Yet I was just happy to let work take over and miss so many games. Which meant missing another occasion to exercise, at least. I was just treating myself with a complete lack of respect. Missing out on things that I love. What is the point in that?

Everywhere you turn now there is a coach or guru telling you that you need to be disciplined with yourself and make sacrifices if you really want to be successful. Sure, sacrifice watching television every night and do something for personal growth, but by no means sacrifice anything that you love.

We still think that we need to trade certain things off in our lives. How very few people actually realise that not only can they have anything in life they want but also just how effortless it can be to achieve it. So many entrepreneurs are still stuck in this mindset, putting everything on hold for a few years then hoping to reap the rewards.

Something that really makes me chuckle is how all of these so-called successful entrepreneurs and coaches out there with millions in the bank tell you to sacrifice your health – albeit indirectly. They tell you that you need to work all the hours under the sun to be successful.

I went through a phase of waking up at 5am for a period of two weeks to see how I would fare. I loved being up early because it made me feel productive. It made me feel proud I had the drive and determination to succeed. What I was oblivious too was how it was affecting other areas.

Not once in those two weeks did I exercise because I was low on energy. Not one day consisted of completely healthy food. And most important of all, I looked dreadful. I only noticed how drained I looked when I was creating a video for YouTube. I am supposed to promote good healthy living and energy whilst looking awful.

Now I have a lot more clarity in what I am doing with my business and having taken greater control of my nutrition and exercise I have so much more energy than before. This has enabled me to get up at 5am feeling a lot fresher and more energised than I did during the first attempt. I wake up with more excitement now and am ready to start my day.

My original experiment was just for two weeks, but erratic sleep patterns were a constant in the initial stages of my time as a business owner. If after three years of doing this all I got was a poor diet, reduced fitness levels and mountain of stress, think what it

Step Five – Madness

would be like if I added another 10 years. Or even 15. That is the position my clients are often in when they come to me.

What I have observed in myself, in my clients and in so many entrepreneurs and small business owners is that we do not take stock of how far we have come. We do not congratulate ourselves for our ever-growing success. Instead, we focus too much on the big goal of all the millions and feel bad about ourselves for not being there yet.

We can work ourselves into the ground for three years, 10 years, 20 years, but it will never bring us success. This is because it is just a constant battle. Wondering why we have not achieved what we wanted to. Becoming accustomed to this way of living and just accepting it as the norm.

Times have changed and we can access any part of the world we want to, be it physically or virtually. We can work whatever hours we want to work. We can create whatever social circles we want and live whatever life we wish. So why are many people stuck working away all the hours under the sun?

I believe we are here for growth and to experience new things. However, I do not believe we are doing enough of it. We all know that life is too short, but it is about maximising every waking second of it. Getting the absolute most out of every situation.

I got to the point where I needed to take action in my life and my work. No longer could I keep chasing success, wasting money and just getting nowhere. I had to go back to the drawing board and decide what it was I really wanted from life. Turns out that I want to have fun. Of course that is not all I want but ultimately that is me, a fun-loving guy.

I had covered up this guy for so long that I forgot he even existed. He was hidden away deep inside me and had no chance to express himself like he used to. I believe that this was what held me back in my pursuit of success. I was not letting the real me come to the fore and was living and acting in a way that felt fake and in no way authentic.

The business world is changing. No longer will buying decisions be made on how well something is sold. We are slowly starting to see past people's intentions and what they want from us. Over the next few years buying decisions will be based on how much someone loves what they do. How transparent they are with their true self and how open they are.

The key word is **authenticity**. How real someone is. We are becoming too clever for the fake people out there who just want to make a quick buck, and we will only spend our money with those who inspire us. As the business owner, we will never have to sell ever again. Prospects will come pre-sold and ready to go.

Step Five – Madness

Everything is exposed now. There is no hiding place. Sure, people buy people, as the saying goes. However, what we will experience going forward is the fact that people buy the right people for them. They will buy the story that resonates with them the most. This is the future of business and there is no escaping that.

How do I know this? I have two examples about myself as both the consumer and the businessman. These were how I truly discovered the way business will be done in the future. There will be many old-school entrepreneurs and business owners out there who will want me to hang for this belief but like anything in life, the truth always comes out eventually.

The first example is me as the consumer. I noticed from Facebook that I had several mutual friends with Elite Life Coach and now author of *A Path To Wisdom*, Tony J Selimi. His profile kept popping up in the section referring to the people I may know. I decided to add him because his profile picture painted a thousand words.

At this point I had no idea what he did. I had not even read anything on his profile or looked for him on other social networking platforms. All I knew was that I needed to add him on Facebook and befriend him. His profile picture was of him on the beach with a huge smile on his face. The kind of smile that told the world just how much he was loving life.

This picture alone resonated with me more than I could explain at the time. It was a gut feeling that I needed to understand what this guy was doing in his life that not only made him so happy but also made him have the huge hunger and zest for life I no longer had. I had already put him on a pedestal based on one single picture. There was something that just felt right.

Despite this, however, I never actually made any contact with him after he had accepted my friend request, but a few weeks later we met at our friend's book launch. I noticed him as soon as he walked through the door and soon he came over to introduce himself.

I finally asked him what he did, and learnt he was a life coach. I was fascinated. So many of my Personal Trainer peers claim to be life coaches but in all honesty, Tony was above and beyond anyone I had met. I kept asking him so many questions about what he did and knew that I needed to find out even more.

The next day I messaged him to book in for a consultation. I felt a great relief come over me, knowing that everything was going to be OK. It was a great feeling and one that I will never forget. Also, I was right to trust my instincts, as the growth I have experienced throughout our coaching has gone far beyond my expectations.

It is important to point out again that all of this came as a result of a solitary picture from Facebook. I did not realise it at the time, but the smile he had in that picture was a result of him living in congruence with his core values. That is what made him so happy and able to enjoy life so much. That is what resonated with me immediately as the consumer. He did not sell anything to me at all. I was pre-sold by the way he lives his life.

The second example is of how I, as a fun loving businessman, came to make a very important discovery. I recently went away to Cyprus for my friend's wedding. I was trusted to be best man and the excitement had been building for quite some time.

I originally planned to go for seven nights and had booked early in the year, but I realised that I needed to be back in London a day earlier so I changed my flight. I was now only to be there for six nights in total – not a long time at all in the grand scheme of things.

I was determined to make the most of every second we had out there and ensure that I had as much fun as I possibly could. Much like when I was in Australia, I was adamant that I would leave no stone unturned.

It is always great to meet new people, especially in a stress-free and fun loving environment. Of course there were a few drunken nights, it was a wedding after all and I was on holiday. Plenty of karaoke would have us laughing all night, then again the following day when reminiscing. Joking around the pool, telling stories. The laughter was non-stop.

Lots of high octane thrills in the sea with speed boats and jet skis. Hitting waves at full throttle and racing around. Quad biking up into the mountains and seeing new parts of the world. Treating oneself to a massage overlooking the sea. Enjoying every second our time there. Having so much fun.

Upon my return home, I had five new sources of income, out of nowhere. I had not so much as looked at my phone while I was away. Made no contact with anyone back home and cut myself off from the working world completely. Five!

This told me one thing. Being my true, authentic, fun-loving self brings me whatever I want in life. It really is as simple as that. I firmly believe that what holds people back and what held me back is the constant pressure we place on ourselves to succeed without even knowing what we are trying to succeed in or why we want to succeed at all.

When I am having fun, things open up for me. That has always been the case, but it took me 29 years to figure it out. When I smile and laugh, I believe the universe rewards me. Purely because I am being authentic to my true self. I am a happy-go-lucky guy with a zest for living and enjoying life.

That zest disappeared when I tried to get what I already had. My social life went, which meant I had no opportunity to laugh. I was not experiencing new things, which meant I could not grow as a person. I could not enjoy what life has to offer. I am a big believer that laughter is the best medicine. I believe that how we feel in ourselves based on important factors such as fun and social interaction can have a huge effect on our immune system.

Society dictates a certain path for us. Sure, as entrepreneurs we ignore some of that path but will still get caught up in other stuff that stops us being who we really are. I observe so much one-upmanship in the entrepreneurial world. Leave all that to the boys in the City. You have at your disposal the most powerful gift of all: your own diary. Do something enjoyable with it.

I would fill up my diary with so many work-related things that I was scheduling 'fun' at least six weeks in advance. Which made it no fun at all. It also gave me the chance to put it so far into the distance that I was not even interested in it by the time it came round. I was missing one very important part of life. Spontaneity.

When was the last time you had a completely random adventure? When was the last time you had a really good laugh? When was the last time you had not a care in the world? There are things in life that we can do nothing about. Therefore stop worrying about them. There are things in life that we can do something about. So do what needs to be done.

Life really is there to be lived. I can pretty much guarantee that you will only regret it later in life if you do not live the way you want to.

Remove the fear of judgement that others may have of you. Why would you even care what others think? I stand by what I said earlier: hard work does not work. At least not when you do not play hard.

EIGHT
Bring It All Together

"I always wonder why birds stay in the same place when they can fly anywhere on earth. Then I ask myself the same question."

HARUN YAHYA

Meaning

Values is a word that gets thrown around too often without people even knowing why or how it is important. It is very easy to pick from a list of character traits and decide that they are your values, but they may be just what society expects from you. We are expected to have honesty and integrity but that does not necessarily paint the full picture of us.

On my own journey of trying to ascertain my values I picked 10 values from a list that seemed to me to be most relevant to my life. Integrity was one of them. Freedom was another. I even used online platforms to pair all my 'values' off against each other to find out what came out on top and to see the hierarchy they form.

What I found was that I was telling myself what I wanted to hear all the time: that I am not interested in money and that I really value my health. I was structuring my answers in a way that would be expected of a Personal Trainer. That was my biggest mistake because I was subordinating myself to the perceived ideology of an entire industry rather than my own personal one.

It was not until I read *The Values Factor* by Dr John Demartini and started looking into *Axiology*, the study of value and self worth, as well as coaching with Tony, that I really started to understand how to determine what my values were. I found it to be a much more in depth process than my previous attempts and started to uncover a lot of hidden truths within myself.

I looked at how I spent my time. What I spent my money on. What really inspired me. What holds my attention the longest. Where and when I am most energetic. What fills up my personal space. What thoughts I have and what I visualise. What areas of my life have organisation. Where I am most reliable. I started to develop a very clear understanding of myself.

It may shock you, given that I work in health and fitness, but **health**, as a value of mine, sits at number four in my hierarchy. And for very good reason. It has never been a major void in my life. Sure I have abused it with binge drinking and sugar over the years, but I have never had any health scares or issues. I value it simply because I fear what losing it may bring.

Bring It All Together

You will often find that your biggest values are a result of your biggest voids. What do you perceive to be lacking in your life that creates a negative emotion? It could be genuine or it could be just a perception. For example, my second value is money. I know I say that chasing it can impact our health but I have a clear understanding as to why it is one of my core values.

Having never had a good relationship with money, it was only a matter of time until I got myself into trouble. I have wasted so much money over the years but it has taught me one hell of a lesson; a lesson that I believe will make me extremely wealthy in the future. I am of course referring to debt.

Spending money on credit cards is a very easy way to abuse our relationship with money. Sooner or later it will catch up with us. I got to a point where I could no longer access credit and it meant having to change the way I dealt with money. Money very quickly became a major void in my life. I had to learn how to cut costs in my business and personal life, how to set monthly and weekly budgets for myself and how to create a pot of savings that does not get touched in any circumstances.

Improving my relationship with money and valuing it more has helped me let go of the *need* to make it. I now trust that it will come. All because I honour my core values, with money being one of them. There is nothing wrong with chasing money, just so long as you know why you are chasing it. Without knowing the reasons why you will just create stress for yourself and step over other people in the process. This can ultimately lead to poor health later in life. You may say that you know why and cite lifestyle and freedom as examples, but until you know why you want that lifestyle and freedom you are putting yourself at risk.

I was not using my credit cards to have a big spend up when I felt like it. I used them to put myself on various workshops and training programmes, both for business and health related topics. Therefore I do view the debt I accumulated as investments but that did not take away the stress I had created for myself.

However, one thing I learned was why I kept spending so much on all these courses. The answer was simple, and subsequently my number one value which is **learning**. Knowledge and education have been the biggest void in my life as a result of how I felt growing up. I believed I did not possess any academic ability and therefore gave up on education before I even started.

On the first day of my Personal Training course I was immediately inspired. It all just clicked. I was fascinated with anatomy, physiology, nutrition and coaching. I was able to retain vast amounts of information. At the time of writing this book I have been a Personal Trainer for four years yet I constantly study because it inspires me. So much so that I meet people that have been in my industry for over 20 years who have only a fraction of the knowledge I have. I say that not to brag but to demonstrate that because **learning** is my number one value, I am inspired to honour it constantly.

This has helped me build confidence in my brain power and my ability to be astute. Aside from the typical subjects a Personal Trainer studies, I have found myself learning on a much deeper level. Subjects such as spirituality, neurophysiology and quantum physics, to name but a few. Mind blowing stuff, but I have had to re-engineer my self-image to develop the belief that I am actually intelligent.

When I wanted to pursue greater success in order to satisfy my childhood desire to prove people wrong, I ended up going overboard and got into debt. Thus creating the void of **money**. Working hard and only able to spend little created a void in my social life which means that **fun** now sits proudly in third place in my hierarchy of values.

They make the top three because they have been my biggest voids in life to date. **Health** sits at number four because of the *fear* of losing it rather than having lost it in some way. Making up my core five values is **teaching**. This is where I am most animated. Whether it be educating a client on something that I have learned, teaching my class of Personal Trainers about how to develop their business, or writing this and other books, I love sharing with people the things that I have learned that can help improve their lives in some way. It is what makes me feel alive.

So now it is time for you to decide what your core values are. What are the biggest voids in your life to date? What do you need to change in your life and why? What do you spend your time and money on? Take your time with this subject. I rushed trying to figure out mine which just wasted my time in the long run. Think carefully and pay attention to everything around you. When you value yourself, so too does everyone else.

Movement

Health is probably one your core values, otherwise you would not be reading this book. We have this value covered in the next two sections and will outline how you can honour this fully. It all starts, as you now know, with physical activity. Getting up and getting moving.

I am not a conventional Personal Trainer. In my view, exercise and diet can merely paper over the cracks of deeper lying issues. During consultations with clients I take them through a comprehensive movement screen. This highlights any imbalances in the body which if not dealt with could lead to injury during exercise.

Contrary to popular belief, poor posture is not necessarily the cause of pain; it is quite often the effect. It may be that there is no pain being experienced at all yet posture is less than desirable. The way I see it is that with poor posture and faulty movement mechanics, exercise efficiency is greatly reduced. In essence, the body has to find a way to carry out a movement and may need to 'steal' it from other areas. Which in turn means that you will fatigue far quicker than is necessary.

As stated earlier, the four key components of achieving true fitness are **variety, enjoyment, strength** and **competition**. I would advise addressing these components in that order and for very good reason. I would have to take you through my extensive movement screen to know if you are very injured, carry a bit of a knock or have absolutely nothing wrong with you.

Given this, I believe it is best to play it safe and get you into a mixture of different sports and activities you can do at your own pace and at your own ability. If you are sedentary for large parts of the day and only go through limited motion, I believe it is best to start off with some variety. This will help to recreate movement patterns of old and can help with overcoming pain or avoid the risk altogether. However, I must state again that as I am unable to watch how you move, any activity you undertake is at your own risk.

Create a list of five different sports and activities. Now put them in order of how enjoyable they are to you and pick the top two to start with. Enjoyment is extremely important. You will not be consistent if you do not like it. For example, running used to bore the absolute life out of me so I would not run as much as I would play football. I see a huge value in running in terms of how good it makes us feel afterwards, but I would not be heartbroken if I missed it.

Now that you have the activities you love, you will most likely need a team or at least a partner to participate with. If you love playing football then you will need to go out and find enough people so that you can play five-a-side with each other every week. If it is squash you enjoy, then you will need a partner to play with. Once you have all these people in place, set a time in your planner, the same time, same day, every week.

This is all about consistency. It also means that no one will let you down. Having a group of people waiting for you will mean that you will never miss a session. Your training will be regular, and it will be enjoyable. Not only that, but a little bit of banter here and there is always welcome.

Now things are starting to get serious. Your fitness levels are up and you want to take things to the next level. This is where the strength component comes in. Again, you may benefit from having a gym buddy so make sure you pick wisely. Someone who is reliable and someone as determined as you are.

When it comes to gym training, I personally want to be in and out in double quick time. I am not a believer in doing short workouts at high intensity because they are typically executed very poorly. I am talking about aiming for maximum strength here. You get the cardio effect from your other activities. This is about lifting heavy weights.

There are plenty of strength exercises we can do in the gym. What we are focused on are the exercises that involve using a lot of big muscle groups. You are aiming for two workouts per week and you can choose any exercises from the following list:

Conventional Deadlift, Sumo Deadlift, Goblet Squat, Front Squat, Back Squat, Barbell Bench Press, Dumbbell Bench Press, Barbell Overhead Press, Dumbbell Overhead Press, Walking Lunges, Reverse Lunges, Step-ups, Pull-ups, Chin-ups, Push-ups, Supine Rows, Rollouts, Pallof Hold, Single Arm Farmers Walk.

Over the course of two sessions per week you will be aiming to cover around five or six exercises in total. This is about aiming for maximum strength but at the start it is important to keep the reps high and the weight low as you work on your technique. Start off with three sets of 12 reps to begin with in the first 30 days. In the second 30 days go down to four sets of eight reps and the final 30 days you will be going for five or more sets of three to five reps. This is just a guide.

It is important to acknowledge the speed of the exercise, known as the tempo. Count for two to four seconds on the way down. This is known as the eccentric phase whereby you are lowing under tension. This creates a better response in terms of building strength and lean muscle as opposed to just rushing. It is also important to stick to appropriate rest times. In phase one, go for 30 to 60 seconds rest between sets. Phase two: one to two minutes. And phase three, up to three minutes. Again, this is just a guide, but a good point to start from.

The exercises above will help you build a solid foundation of strength which will not only reduce risk of injury, if executed in good form, but will also improve your performance in your chosen sports and activities.

Now we move onto the super serious business of competition. This is where you sign yourself up for some kind of event or race. It may be a 10km run. It may be a strongman competition. You may even get your group together and set up a football tournament one day.

The point is that you will really be able to test yourself to see how far you have come. You will be able to push yourself more than you would do not only by yourself but in your group settings as well. For example, when I go to football training and we have five-a-side matches and specific drills, though it is obviously challenging, it is very difficult to replicate the tempo of a competitive game in the league. In the game, where there is something riding on it, you are more inclined to give it your maximum.

The same can be said for a long distance running event. Running out by yourself or with a partner or group is great. You will certainly benefit a great deal from it because it still very much counts as exercise. However, a race is a race. And you want to win it!

Mindful Meals

As I've mentioned, exercise and diet are often required as a result of some deeper issues. If eating has gotten you to a point where you are carrying more weight than you want, or you lack adequate energy, or both, then there is a reason why you rely on it. It fills some kind of void that you need to get to the bottom of. It is satisfying a unconscious need.

For example, I find comfort in food when I am tired, stressed and have no social interaction. It is my body's way of telling me that it needs some 'goodness'; that I need to make some changes to my diary!

I am not the type of Personal Trainer who gives out meal plans and quick and easy diet strategies. I am a Personal Trainer who looks way beyond the superficial to teach my clients how to learn about themselves. This, I believe yields greater and sustainable results. Sure, I could create meal plans for clients and they would have instant success. Motivation would be high and everything great. Then an episode flares up: work, family, whatever it may be, and all of a sudden we go back to square one because the focus was lost.

The better you get to know yourself, the better you will become at handling any situation that is thrown at you. You will become more in tune with your body and will be able to plan accordingly when and if something arises. It is all well and good me telling someone what to eat, but without them knowing why it will be no different to a yo-yo diet. I see myself more as an educator than a trainer. However, there are the basics of nutrition that, when habitual, can make a massive difference to overall health and energy.

When it comes to nutrition, you will need to be a little bit clever and think outside the box. The way I coach my clients, and now you, the reader, is first to look at the first 30 days of a 90-day plan and see what engagements you have coming up. Are you going to a special birthday party? Have you got a wedding reception to go to? These occasions in particular will mean that you are more than likely to drink and help yourself to a slice or three of cake.

I do not begrudge anybody of this type of enjoyment. I do, however, look at damage limitation and where we can offset the temporary indulgence. We are only human and there is no way that anyone should be made to miss out all the time. Although considerable effort will need to be made elsewhere.

Once you have your particular celebratory events in place in your first 30 days you will need to count them up. Then decide if that is too many. In this day and age it is any excuse so some common sense would need to be applied here. Two or three occasions is ample. Any more than that and you are on the water, pal!

The next step is to fill out a food diary for the first seven of your 90 days. Be completely honest and include the time of consumption as well as mood. Be sure to include liquids on the diary too: water, coffee, alcohol…

At the end of the week, go back over the food diary and highlight what you believe to be the bad selections then pinpoint what your decision was based on. As I mentioned earlier, it could be stress that had you reaching for the sugar treats. It could be tiredness that got you reaching for the comfort foods. This was usually my pattern.

Having understood what the driver was, you are now able to carry out a risk assessment to ensure limited impact next time round. For example, if it was down to tiredness then how can you avoid getting up at a time that does not suit you? Can you push meetings back? If it was a lunch meeting with a client, ensure you order the healthiest thing on the menu next time. It will impress your client!

There is always a way to overcome these stumbling blocks. It is mainly a question of raising your awareness to your decision-making. Understanding what led you to that decision in the first place will make it a whole lot easier to manage and avoid going forward. Your body has infinite wisdom; it knows what it wants. The key is in cleaning up that link between body and mind.

The next step when it comes to nutrition is busting a few of the myths my industry has thrown at you in recent years. Firstly, there is no right way to eat. Sure, there are particular diets out there which will work for some, and other diets that will work for others.

However, as I mentioned, your body knows what it wants. Treat yourself well and you will naturally seek better quality foods.

The idea that you need '200g' of this and '150ml' of that is a model that you may have followed up until now. Also, the idea that you need to eat a certain number of meals each day and at particular times can be quite vague as we are all very different. However, there are certain things that will help toward boosting your energy, improving your outlook and making that food diary look awesome.

Hydration is vitally important. And one that I take for granted in people because I am always attached to a bottle of water. I have never tasted coffee in my life! I am always surprised when people tell me they do not drink a great deal of water. If I have anything less than two litres each day, I feel incredibly groggy.

Coffee-drinkers go for the caffeine hit for the short-term energy boost. Therefore, keeping on top of exercise and nutrition will ensure optimal energy anyway which should render coffee unnecessary. Having never even tasted it perhaps I have no idea, but I would strongly suggest you look at cutting down and eventually giving it up. You really do not need it.

Good quality hydration will help you think clearly as well as keeping you alert. It is a massively overlooked component of good health. Be sure to drink at least two litres each day of quality mineral water. In fact, whenever I first see a client with low back pain, the first thing

I get them to do is increase their water intake. Our discs will rehydrate throughout the night so without adequate hydration our spine cannot function as best as it can. You will be surprised at how effective this simple tip can be.

One habit I got myself in is to squeeze a lemon into a pint of chilled water first thing every morning. There is a belief that the water needs to be lukewarm, but chilled lemon water certainly wakes you up!

Next up we have **fresh produce**. The government will tell you to eat five fruits and veg each day. In fact I believe that they have now upped it to seven. However, we are rebels against society so we do not listen to the government. Make it a minimum of 10, then. And that is just for veg! In all honesty I like to aim for around 20.

It does make me laugh whenever I get resistance on even the five a day. It really is not that hard. You can get at least five into a juice. If you plan to have something green with every meal then you can really clock them up. Another myth is that eating healthily is expensive. Then again, so is alcohol. So is dining out. So are takeaways.

If you struggle with a sweet tooth, fruit can be a good substitute. It has worked really well for me. Two or three pieces per day will suffice to help take that edge off. More often than not I will have a banana straight after a workout.

I personally gave up meat and fish a while back. I am not suggesting that you do the same because different things work for different people. My energy levels have gone through the roof and I do not feel sluggish in any way at all, as I used to. I feel much better as a result. For others, meat is an essential part of their diet. Your job is to ascertain how you feel after eating certain things.

Ensure that you consume the best quality meats and fish there are. Purchase from farmers markets as opposed to supermarkets. Supermarkets sell meat from animals that have not necessarily been well-treated, and have very poor standards when it comes to quality. Ideally aim for organic. You will also be supporting small business, so everyone's a winner.

The final myth I will cover is that healthy food takes an age to prepare. Wrong again. I would always use this excuse, but quite frankly I was lazy. Sure it would be easier for me to grab something while I was out than it would be put a meal together, but I soon realised that there was not a great deal of difference.

Realistically, how long does it take to put together a salad consisting of spinach, cucumber, celery, olives, tomatoes and whatever else you want to throw in. Add in a chopped up avocado, some pine nuts, drizzle some olive oil over it. Pre-prepare a green juice when making it and you are killing two birds with one stone. You would also have easily hit your target of 10 vegetables for the day. It really is that simple; sometimes it is more about lack of responsibility than a lack of time.

I do not eat a great deal of dairy: some cheese now and then, but milk does not sit right with me so I will have almond milk or rice milk as a substitute. I also find that gluten products affect my digestion. Therefore I will avoid breads and instead get my starchy carbs in the form of quinoa, kidney beans and buckwheat which also have a decent amount of protein in for us vegetarians. I also love a sweet potato quite regularly. Starchy foods give us the energy to exercise at a high intensity.

Fat still has a bad reputation despite the overwhelming evidence that it is actually good for you. Of course not all fat is good for you. For example, you want to avoid the trans-fats and hydrogenated fats that are typically found in vegetable based products, believe it or not. Fats to incorporate in your diet are oils such as olive oil for salads and coconut oil for cooking. Nuts and seeds. Avocados, despite them not tasting very nice. Apparently I am on my own with that one! The good fats will help with your energy.

The key is **energy**. You do not want to feel sluggish. You want to be bouncing off the walls with optimum vitality. This involves committing to looking after yourself as well as tuning into your body to see what it needs and what it wants. Understanding why that is so and acting accordingly.

With cleaner nutrition, as described above, you will naturally have a higher intake of fibre which will assist in optimising your digestive system. The digestive system goes through a constant battle when we bombard it with junk food. I would encourage a diet whereby over half of it is raw. This is because raw foods have within them their own digestive enzymes which means they do not require the digestive system to help out as much as it would with cooked food.

This in turn means that our stomach acids do not take as long to replenish, which again is a big job for our bodies. Not all raw food necessarily works this way. For example, nuts and seeds require you to soak them overnight in order to unlock their own digestive enzymes. Having plenty of raw vegetables in the form of a juice or a salad, along with some fruit each day, should suffice in this quest.

Nothing I am telling you here is new information. You know what is good and bad for you. You just need to control the driver. This is not a new diet fad, nor will I promote such a thing. This is about getting the basics right and building a solid foundation and awareness to the nutritional approach that is right for you.

Managing Time

I dread to think how much time I have haemorrhaged over the years on pointless tasks that really amounted to nothing. It is all a learning curve, of course, but time is always ticking and something we never get back. It is about time that we showed time more respect and made the absolute most of it. We all know that life is too short, but we also find it incredibly easy to just let time sail by in the blink of an eye.

When Steve Jobs was diagnosed with his terminal illness he pointed out that we will all die one day and that when he accepted that, he let go of any fears that he had throughout his life. Though he was already a major success, he was still able to put everything into perspective.

Using my example of my Cyprus holiday, making the most of every second made me feel on top of the world. I really cannot explain just how good it felt to maximise my time. I have also experienced the other side of the coin when I would waste time and feel awful about it.

This is how I know I value time. When I do not honour it, I feel bad. I feel that time is always running out and if I just let it sail by I get angry and frustrated. On so many occasions we let our time be dictated by others and so completely neglect the time we need for ourselves.

I am not saying you should not help others in any way. Not at all. What I am saying is that it needs to be your decision. You decide how you will spend your time. You will decide how you commit to helping people. Once you put it in your terms and respect yourself for it, you will automatically get respect from others as a result.

In the business world this happens every minute of every day. I am of course talking about email. I spent far too much time checking my emails and realised that I was not actually getting much work done.

I could have been writing, I could have been learning something new or I could have been exercising. Of course, for many of you reading this, email is a hugely important part of your business. However, are you spending more time than is necessary using it?

I challenge you to calculate the amount of time you spend on email every day. It will equate to hours! How better could you spend some of that time? What important tasks are you putting off as a result of checking email?

Reading and responding to an email may only take a minute. Multiply that by how many emails you typically receive in a day, week, month, year. Now ask yourself: were *all* of those emails of high priority? Are you able to separate high value tasks from low values ones?

Another way to waste time is social media. Of course, I am on all the platforms but I dread to think how much time I have wasted going through news feeds and checking notifications when I could have put that time to better use. I would spend so much time clicking on Facebook, Twitter and LinkedIn at least 20 times a day each. That probably equated to at least a couple of hours every day: time that, again, could have been spent reading, writing, exercising or preparing healthier meals.

I decided to take drastic action and went down to checking them all once per day. This made a huge difference. I would still spend a fair amount of time on them, although considerably less than before. So I took further action and decided to just check notifications, which I soon discovered were not all that important to me in many cases. I do not really need to know if some 'likes' my updates.

At one stage I even deleted all the apps from my iPhone. I realised something even more powerful when it came to time management: not only was I saving much more time and getting more things done, but I was also thinking more clearly and creating better content, such as e-books and actually getting down to write this book.

I believe that this is because I was not filling my head with low value content for those few hours each day from people's status updates and shared links. I was not allowing nonsense to get into my brain and cloud my thinking. My mind felt freer and was able to better access my own wisdom as a result of less consumption.

Everywhere you turn there is information overload. We cannot escape it. I was so attached to my phone that I might as well have had it surgically implanted. It is as if we cannot get enough. We need to know everything and we need to know it now. Right this second.

For quite a few years now I have not bothered watching or reading any news. I just believe that it is all fabricated. For me, it is no more real than a soap opera! So why bother? And talking of trashy television, is that something that you want to consume as well? Or magazines filled with rubbish?

Become an expert in how you spend your time. None of that junk brings you any value. All it does is clutter your brain. It stops your creative juices from flowing and puts you right back where the rest of society wants you. A place that keeps you living in fear and keeps you living small time. When it comes to consumption, read some inspiring books, explore the arts or watch educational documentaries. Something, anything, that will help you grow. The news, television, and all that stuff will shrink you.

Another thing I found that I wasted my time with were so many networking events. I do believe that there are some great events out there and I have been to a few. On the whole, though, they only work for people who turn up with an agenda, people who want to sell you something and have no interest in what you do. Be sure to work out what events will be valuable to you and which are a waste of time.

I am a firm believer that if you make time for the truly important things in life then you will excel in time management. This is purely because you will not have the time to be spending doing the things you do not want to do. What many fail to realise is that this is a unique time in our existence where we no longer have to do anything we do not want to.

It often amuses me when entrepreneurs tell me that they need to get better at time management or at saving time so they can free time up for important things. I just believe that this is the complete opposite of how to actually achieve the life that we all want. Just do what you want to do and everything will work out nicely.

Managing Stress

Doing what you want to do will remove so much stress from your life. You are free to do anything that you desire. You can let go of judgment from other people and just be your authentic and true self. You would not even know the meaning of the word stress.

Of course there are several other ways to beat stress and for me personally, one way that is way up there is putting everything into perspective. Sometimes it really does astound me just how lucky we are and just how oblivious we are to that luck. That is because I was completely oblivious to it.

Back in 2008 and 2009 there was the banking crisis which led to a recession. I was on the other side of the world having a whale of a time so I had no idea. I did try to catch up on it all but soon got bored of listening to people moaning about nonsense. Upon returning home from Australia, I noticed a lot of new cars on the road. It must not have been that bad. I expected to see boarded up buildings and tumbleweed everywhere!

Consumerism has such a stranglehold on society that nowadays a recession is defined as having to shop in Sainsbury's rather than Waitrose. I thought recessions were about people not being able to eat at all. Of course for some people that may have been true, and many were hit extremely hard, but the people who moaned the most appeared to be the people who already had so much.

It beggars belief why we cannot see just how fortunate we are. Especially in Britain. The amount of opportunity we have here and what we can achieve is amazing. It is a fantastic country and one that I know I am extremely lucky to live in.

My Australian experience means I see myself as a citizen of the world rather than a particular nationality, but to be able to call England home is a real honour. What troubles me, though, is just how people rush around London, barging people out of the way on the tube, complaining that trains are delayed. There always seems to be some kind of injustice for some people.

Let me tell you, I was one of these people, getting so worked up, angry and frustrated over the smallest of things. This is a great way to get stressed. Everything annoyed me. Everything. I would have mental arguments with people in my head because I thought something might kick off somewhere. Looking back, I realise that I was just not very loving at all, to myself or to the rest of humanity.

Bring It All Together

When we let go of the control we feel at peace. We try to control situations such as train delays and queues by moaning about them. Not only will that not fix the situation, not only will it stress you out, but it will also make the situation feel worse. The universe gives back what you put out there. Increasing your negative vibration will only send it straight back.

What really is the worst that can happen? You are late for a meeting? Sure, we have established that you value the time of yourself and of others, but if something is beyond your control then what can you do about it? Nothing. We are more understanding than we make out to be. Chill out, this sort of thing is not life threatening.

As I mentioned earlier, **perspective**. Very few people in the world have as much as you have. They get by and just get on with it. Grateful to be alive. When you stop trying to control things out of your power you will soon find that you get closer to inner peace. You are calmer and you can think a lot more clearly.

This goes hand in hand with **acceptance**. Accepting situations, accepting people. Just let what will be, be. Nothing is worth getting worked up over. There really is no point. If there is something you do not like or agree with, just remove yourself from the situation. Let others carry on as they are.

The best way to inspire people is to be your best self. If this resonates with someone, they will ask for your help or guidance.

Trying to force your ideology on people will leave you frustrated and them alienated. This is why sales will soon be a thing of the past. Selling is a dead duck. There is no place for it in the new economy. People will see right through it.

I used to put an extreme amount of pressure on myself to be super successful and make millions upon millions. I guess I was scared that it would run out. The idea of accumulation is stressful. My coach, Tony, always makes a very good point that we cannot take anything with us when we go. He taught me that if we have infinite wisdom within us, why do we need so much "stuff" *around* us?

Putting pressure on ourselves to accumulate wealth just breeds stress. As I stated earlier, when I let go of the need to make money, I ended up making more. This is because we were previously giving our attention to perceived scarcity. You still have a roof over your head, food on the table and great people around you. What more could you ask for in life?

Sometimes we really need to take a step back and appreciate just how lucky we are to have what we already have and be grateful. This is what will bring you more and will calm down the perceived stresses in life. Nothing in life is worth getting stressed over. If you can fix something then fix it. Stress gone. If you cannot control something then do not worry about it. Stress gone. Chill out and smile. That will fix everything!

Madness

I have said it before; I will say it again. Life is too short. Have more fun, laugh more, experience more new things. Bring back that busy social life from days gone by. Work can wait. In fact, you will be more productive as a result. **Social interaction** makes us feel good. It makes us happier and therefore more able to focus on our projects.

Being an entrepreneur can be a lonely place. I work from home some days and even though I am busy creating content and getting on with important tasks, I still crave social interaction. We are social beings, after all. We are meant to connect and laugh and enjoy each other's energy. Working hard in my business ended up with my social life evaporating completely.

I knew I needed to change something because there was no way I could carry on as I was. I was getting more and more miserable by the day. Devoting all my time to trying to become successful just meant that I was moving further away from what success actually is.

With a conscious effort to make more time to go out with friends, I gradually started to pull my social life back. From the ages of 25-28 I did nothing with my life other than work. Sure, I gained a lot of experience from it. It gave me a story to tell and helped me develop my coaching practice based on my work with clients and my own mistakes. However, I cannot help but think I missed out on so many things in that time.

I believe that a social life is a vitally important component of health and, of course, success. It can get completely overlooked in favour of continuous work.

In order to inspire others you need to be your best self. Working all the hours under the sun sends a message to your offspring that life is hard when in actual fact it can be very easy. I am not saying that you must abandon everything and go out raving just like in the old days. I am saying that you do not have any right to neglect yourself. If you want to have fun, go have fun. Work hard only if you play hard.

During the recession a few years back, three areas that achieved substantial growth were health clubs, short breaks and cinema. This tells us that 'Me' time has finally come back to the fore and is starting to increase in importance. We are putting ourselves back on the map.

Taking the time to focus on ourselves, be it through pampering, meals out with friends, or holidays, means that we forget all the issues we have in business. We take ourselves out of the equation and just have some fun and relax. When we return to work, we are able to apply more creativity and logic to overcome any hurdles. We can think a lot more clearly than before. We have within us all the answers. Having some fun will help us access them quicker.

I make a point of going away a minimum of five times every year. I love travel. I love having fun. I want to experience new things and new cultures. It gives me a big burst of energy when I get back to carry on with my creations. I believe it makes me a better person, a better coach and a better businessman.

When I am away I meet new people. I learn new things. I value people very much. We can learn so much from each other. We can connect with others and share our wisdom and our beliefs. When so many entrepreneurs nowadays are trying to create online businesses, I am creating an offline one.

I have entrepreneurs tell me that they want or have an online business that they can run from anywhere and make money by being completely free. You are already free. You just create traps for yourself. I created a prison for myself by working all the time, cutting myself off from everyone and everything. Stop ignoring the value of human interaction. Entrepreneurship is already a lonely place.

We no longer have that model of work hard for 40 years and enjoy retirement, with freedom to do what you want only coming in the latter stages of one's life. Life is a journey. A trip around the world is about the journey, not necessarily the destination. Why wait to have the life that you want when you already have it in front of you?

Travel helps to reaffirm my belief of how free we all are. I can go away whenever I want and so can you. Virtually everyone I speak to shares my passion for travel. Yet so few people are actually doing it.

One thing that my friends and I do is a secret holiday. We will do two or three each year. We each put money into a kitty and one person is in charge of booking flights and accommodation to somewhere in Europe for a weekend. The rest have no idea where it is until arriving at the airport. No idea what to pack or anything. The spontaneity yields fun, laughter and enjoyment.

You have taken a gamble in life that most could only dream of. You became an entrepreneur. You rebelled against society and you built your passion and your beliefs. That needs to be rewarded. You owe it to yourself to thank yourself for being you. Overcoming obstacles and resistance to be where you are today deserves self-appreciation.

There are entrepreneurs who put super successful entrepreneurs on a pedestal and aspire to be just like them. It would appear that they all want the glory and riches of those like Sir Richard Branson for example. Yet they try to achieve it in completely the opposite way. Branson insists that he would never do anything unless it is going to be fun. Both in business and in life. It was the fun that made it successful. Not the success that made it fun.

NINE
The Application

> "Wisdom is the right application of knowledge; and true education... is the application of knowledge to the development of a noble and Godlike character."
>
> **DAVID O. MCKAY**

Now you have gone through the five key steps and taken on board what I believe to be the most important factors when it comes to business ownership, it is time to start applying it. It is one thing to read something and learn about it but it is a whole other thing to put it into practice. Those who get results are those who apply what they've learned.

I have put the five key steps in this order for a reason. I believe that mastering the first will help you master the next, and the next, and so on. I have come to this conclusion based on my own experience in health and business ownership and that of my clients.

I believe knowing our true meaning will give us clarity and direction in life. With this, we become more conscious of our health for some very important reasons. Notably, we want to enjoy our lives and our calling with abundant energy and vitality, not to mention longevity.

Movement is key when it comes to being productive, having a clearer mind and optimal energy levels. In my experience, and that of my clients, it comes before nutrition. There have been so many occasions in training my clients when they have remarked how they are more inclined to eat better when they are immersed in physical activity.

We end up valuing eating well once we start an exercise regime. Then we ensure that we are preparing and consuming highly nutritious **meals** that aid our training, boost our energy, and enhance our productivity in business.

Now we know what we want from life, and have greater energy as a result of regular exercise and good nutrition we are better equipped to **manage time**. I have been questioned about this idea, typically by people with no concept of how to manage their time effectively. They will say that it all starts with time management because we can fit exercise and meal preparation around our working week.

This is flawed logic because if that were the case then everyone would do it. The fact is, we *make* time to exercise and prepare healthy meals. Everything else can fit in around that. It does not take second place to work. Not any more. It takes equal importance.

I mentioned in the last chapter that consumers will see past all the bravado. That also goes for how well we look after ourselves.

I refuse point blank to spend my money with anyone who has no desire to take care of themselves. You are your business; your business is a mirror image of you. If you do not make yourself a priority and ensure that you love and value yourself then you will come up short in the new economy.

Now that we have fixed time in our diary to ensure we stay fit and healthy, we know what time we have for working. Now we can start to be picky with our choices. We can decide what tasks create the most value and focus solely on them. Getting quicker and more productive in doing the menial tasks will only free that time up for more of the same.

We are fitter, we are healthier, we are more productive, we have greater clarity and a sense of direction in our lives. We have become much more content and carefree. So does stress even exist? Sure there may be times when it rears its ugly head. However, do you think you will now be better equipped to handle whatever is thrown at you?

Once you have a clearer mind, reduced tension and greater thinking power, stress soon becomes very manageable indeed. You are able to put things into perspective much more easily than before. Not much will worry you. In fact, you will most likely be amused at what once bothered you.

And finally the **play time**. Is life not so much more enjoyable when you do not have a care in the world? Sure, you could have a very active social life but just how present are you? Sure, you can make time for your family but the same question still applies. With everything ticking over nicely, your mind is free to ensure you have infinite fun when you are meant to. Life is there to be lived to the full, remember. We all need a little bit of **madness** in our lives!

Where To Begin

First you will need to create a 90-day planner. You can do this on a paper or online diary, an Excel spreadsheet or an A3 sheet of paper. We will be working in 30-day blocks with Day One being the preparation and planning day and Day 30 the day to review the previous four weeks.

I would encourage you to go by this 90-day block regardless of when the days fall because it can be very tempting to put off starting until a Monday or the first of the month, for example. All this does is just build up the potential dread of starting something new or having to adapt to change. As far as I am concerned, today is Day One, the planning day and you implement your plan as of tomorrow.

Before you fill out your plan you need to uncover what your core values are. Using the process I described in the previous chapter, take your time to sit down and work out what you value the most. Be it from a place of perceived lack, childhood 'trauma' or changes you want to see in yourself.

For each of your core values, write down three to five ways you can honour them to the best of your ability. For example, as I have mentioned, one of my core values is **money**. It is not my driving force but I have finally learned to respect and honour its power. Having spent so long being frivolous with money and squandering it, I realised that it did not make me feel good about myself.

Now, before the start of each month I write out everything that is due to come out in that month. Both for business and personal. It shows me what I have as disposable income and also highlights areas that I could perhaps cut back on and reduce overall expenditure. I then review this on a weekly basis to ensure that everything is on track.

Another way I honour my value of money is to save a percentage of what I make every month. I just transfer it across to an online savings account and let it build up. It is surprising just how quickly it rises and certainly helps with the anxiety we can often have when it comes to money. It helps us take greater control of money rather than the other way round.

The third way I honour money is to recycle it. At the start of each month, I work out what outgoings can be paid in cash and draw that money out of the bank. As a result there is loose change which I put into a pot. Whenever I need to go to the shop for a bottle of water, for example, I use the coins rather than using my debit card as I always used to. Using our debits cards for the small things is a really easy way to fly through money.

These are three ways I honour my value of money: a monthly basis, a weekly basis and even a daily basis. These work exceptionally well for me and have increased the abundance in my life. I believe that because I am showing money a much greater respect, I am making more. Like they say, look after the pennies and the pounds will look after themselves.

Now that you have your list of core values and the ways in which you will honour them, you are able to look at how they will fit into your planner. You may even change your core values over time, so it is important to go through this process again when you come to your next 90 days.

Now it is time to get **planning**. Taking your 90-day plan, the first thing that goes in is **a holiday.** Reward yourself with a holiday every three months. Go away with friends or family. It can be a short weekend break, it can be a week or even a fortnight. Just make sure you take a break every quarter.

Taking time off at home may not necessarily be a break. I am sure you will find ways of straightening out things whilst periodically checking your email. Get away and go have some fun. That is all you need to focus on. Work will be there when you get back and you will be better equipped to handle it.

The reward is the most important thing to attend to. Now, on to your **health and fitness** goals. By the end of the 90 days do you want your favourite sports to be a regular weekly activity all in full flow? Do you want to have a six pack? Do you want to increase your energy? Get it written down. Not forgetting also what fitness event are you going to compete in in this 90 days?

I mentioned at the start of this book that a large majority of my clients have been male. Regardless of gender, this all applies equally. And not just gender either, it can relate to people of different abilities in health and fitness. The important thing is about getting started and sticking to a plan that is right for you.

Next you need to ask yourself what you want to achieve in business in that 90-day period so that you enjoy your reward as best you can. Do you need to finish a particular project? Do you need a certain number of clients? Whatever it is, write it down.

Now we break it down into three parts. In each of the 30-day blocks you will task yourself with getting certain things done. Are you going to take your partner away at the end of each month for some pampering? Going to have a day out with friends? Figure out the reward first then everything else will fall into place.

How many exercise sessions are you going to get done in the first 30 days? How many healthy meals are you going to prepare? How much time will you look to save on things that bring you no value? How will you ensure that you honour all your values? Can you see a marked improvement in each block compared to the previous 30 days? How can you get better still?

Break it further down on a weekly basis. What meetings do you have this week? Can you make a few back to back? What days will you exercise? What day will you take your family out and leave your phone at home? What day will you go out with friends and leave your phone in your pocket? What will you make yourself for lunch this week?

Now we look at day by day. What time does your body want to wake up and go to sleep? How can you schedule work around that? What time of the day is best for you to exercise? What chunk of time are you going to give to certain projects with full focus to ensure completion? What can you do on a daily basis to honour your values?

These are all questions that you will need to be asking yourself each and every day. First looking at the entire 90 days and deciding what is it that you want to do and achieve in that period; then breaking it all down into smaller and smaller chunks.

You may be reading this and thinking that in an ideal world this can work, but we do not live in an ideal world. My view is that it is down to you to create your ideal world. It does not just happen, it requires going through a process of self-discovery to understand what works best for you. You have to commit to getting to know your body, your mind and your spirit.

TEN
Young At Heart

"We don't stop playing because we grow old; we grow old because we stop playing."

GEORGE BERNARD SHAW

As soon as I came up with the idea for *Move Play Explore*, many people told me to aim for corporates and big companies. All because that is where the money is, apparently. Truth be told, whilst for some people the corporate world may be a way to honour their true values, I personally love the freedom that comes from the entrepreneurial world.

The way we are living our lives, it makes more sense for someone like me to help others who prefer this route. Many are awakening to the fact that their needs and values are not being met in working for companies that place money as the driving force behind everything they do.

I believe in entrepreneurship. I believe that it is the future of our economy. I believe that small businesses can thrive alongside major corporations by moving away from having to compete with one another into a more collaborative environment.

This is because when entrepreneurs, major corporations, and small businesses come together from value driven service they can create a caring community.

Historically, many big corporations have cared only about the amount of money they have been making. This is why I want to help create **Bulletproof Entrepreneurs**, to bring balance, harmony and add more value so that everyone can benefit.

I want to help people who work for themselves because that takes guts, courage and a lot of time. I found it extremely hard to make this transition. We often face oppression from society. By working for ourselves we go in pursuit of a life we want to live and not one dictated to us by anybody else.

We take risks in search of the bigger picture. The bigger picture is that there is a far better world out there compared to the one that is forced upon us right now.

As someone who is heart-driven, what better cause for me to assist in than the health and wellbeing of all entrepreneurs out there who rebel against society's strict and old ideologies that no longer serve a conscious community.

My hope is that helping fun-loving, healthy and happy entrepreneurs live their best lives possible will enable them to inspire others that may be considering breaking free from the nine to five lifestyle. The way I see it right now is that so many entrepreneurs are not living their values, are unable to make a living as they do not really know how to sell their lifestyle very well, nor have the clarity that I have developed through having Tony as my personal coach.

Cutting off the best that life has to offer to immerse ourselves in running a business, having to work longer hours and making less money than the average employee is in no way desirable or inspiring. As entrepreneurs we have within us the key ingredients to live whatever life we want to live, right from the very start. Why toil away for something you already have?

My dream is to create a community of fit and active entrepreneurs who love life. A community of entrepreneurs who value themselves as much as their business. A community of entrepreneurs who want to grow and share their wisdom. A community of entrepreneurs who want to squeeze as much as they possibly can out of life and enjoy it to the full. A community of entrepreneurs who see the sheer amount of value that having fun can bring to the world.

I have another reason for doing what I do. It is a big driver and one that really gets me out of bed every morning. I believe this is the reason for my existence. To help people see just how important a factor it is in living their best lives possible. I am, of course, referring to **never feeling old**. Or perhaps, more appropriately, **always feeling young**.

Since I could walk, I could run. I have always been fit and active. An all-round sportsman who could never sit still. Something I have always taken for granted. Something that I always assumed I would have and would never lose. Coupled with optimum vitality, high energy levels and a real zest for life.

In my time as a Personal Trainer I have had so many clients – again, mostly male in their late 30s or early 40s – who have said how different they felt compared to when they were in their 20s.

At first I would just bat this comment off as a bit of moaning and groaning on their part. Nothing to take any notice of. Why would I? I was as fit as a fiddle. No issues at all. However, things started to hit home a little more. I started to pay attention to what they were saying. Then fear struck right through me. The idea that one day age would hit me like it does everyone else.

For I was one of those business owners going down the same route that my clients had gone down. Missing training sessions, eating bad food, working long hours, losing sleep, being stressed up to the eyeballs. This is how the idea of age kicks in. It has nothing to do with anything else. We allow age to happen to us by the way we treat ourselves.

I found that the decreased activity in my life was helping old football injuries rear their ugly heads. Everything ached. Everything was an effort. I consumed comfort foods as a way to cheer myself up. This left me feeling drained. I had no social life. Another reason to reach for junk food. Every day was Groundhog Day. It was monotonous and boring. I had come so far from that happy-go-lucky young fella high on life.

Endless hours of work is a far cry from the endless hours of play that we experienced in childhood. Society just expects us to carry on along the conveyor belt. We are rebels against this ideology but still insist on keeping ourselves closely attached. Going along with what is deemed acceptable. Still fearing judgement despite making a breakthrough when becoming a business owner.

I am not disputing degeneration when it comes to our bodies ageing. What I am suggesting is that we are going out of our way to accelerate it and then we moan about it. There are plenty of older folk out there competing in marathons and lifting heavy weights in the gym, with no issues whatsoever. Consumerism being what it is nowadays, we sacrifice the important things for the shiny new things.

If you suffer with low back pain or dodgy knees, do you believe it is a sign of age or do you believe that it could have a lot more to do with inactivity? How many injuries did you have when you were a child? Bearing in mind you were bouncing around all over the place and putting yourself at greater risk than you are now.

And **risk** is a very important word. Why have we become so scared in adult life? What are we afraid of? I broke my wrist as a child.

Shattered the bone in three places. When the cast came off I did not even bother with the physiotherapy they advised. I just went back out to play. I have never had an issue since. If we break a limb as an adult we dare not move for so long for fear of doing more damage. It is ironic that the lack of movement increases further injury risk than actually moving.

If we insist on not moving when we are injured just to escape risk of further injury then how can we heal properly? Without adequate blood flow getting to a particular area it will be starved of nutrients, which will slow down the healing process and increase the ageing process.

What about **energy**? As kids we had so much energy. Rushing around all over the place. It was never ending. We had energy to burn back then but now it would appear that that gravy train has reached the terminus. And of course it would have, because in all honesty, dietary habits have not changed enough.

Yes, we are becoming more health conscious, which is great. That does not seem to stop the self-sabotage that occurs so regularly in people. It certainly occurred in me. We can no longer get away with eating the endless amounts of rubbish that we did in our younger days. Our body has become wiser and has a better understanding of what it needs to function optimally.

It has become our responsibility to create that **energy** now, through good quality nutrition. Fuelling our bodies with only what is necessary to ensure we have boundless energy. Giving our bodies the nutrients they need to help us face any obstacle with a clear head and optimal vitality.

What about **time and stress**? As kids we had all the time in the world. Sure we squandered a lot of it, but we did not care. Now we are more aware that time is escaping us so why are we not in a mad dash to enjoy as much of life as possible? What were we doing with our time in our younger years? Having fun. Messing around. Laughing. Playing.

I am not religious, but Jesus once said, "Truly I tell you, unless you change and become like little children, you will never enter the kingdom of heaven." (*Matthew* 18.3) What fantastic words they are. What died in us and turned us into worrying stress freaks? When we were kids we did not have a care in the world. We did not even know the meaning of the word stress. We had not even heard of it.

What about **values**? Life was much simpler then, of course. We valued friendships and social interaction. We valued experiences. We valued fun. We valued laughter. I do not believe that we stopped valuing these things as we moved into adulthood. I believe we stopped honouring them in adulthood, which is why life can feel like such a chore sometimes.

We enter adulthood and create for ourselves all these responsibilities and restrictions, subconsciously, I believe, to detract us from living from our inner child. We blend in with society and shut off what is truly important to us. We fear judgement for being immature so we subordinate ourselves to other people's ideology, all the while taking us further and further away from our authenticity. Further away from our happiness.

I fell into the trap of working hard without playing hard. I fell into the trap of unhappiness that society has created for us. I fell into the trap of thinking that if I made millions then I would be free and happy. This just made me feel more trapped. It did not feel loving to myself in any way.

Happiness is one of the most researched subjects ever. We are falling over ourselves trying to figure out how to be happy. We feel the answer is in material wealth. I am not disputing that money can and does have its advantages. I just believe that doing nothing but chasing it makes us feel bad about ourselves. I also believe that we will make more of it when we stop pursuing it and start to be our authentic selves.

Success will not necessarily make us happy. Yet happiness will certainly make us successful. At this point in time we need to create a new definition of success. One that covers all the key areas in our life. One that is not all about financial accumulation but more about experiences and pleasure.

My theory is that we long to become our childlike selves again. We get so bogged down with the perceived journey of life that matches up with society's plan for us. We fear the judgement of being truly who we are. Being authentic.

The irony is that I embarked on my own journey into entrepreneurship to be successful and to accumulate riches. When I figured out where my passion was and what I wanted out of life, the money mattered a little less and I started making a lot more. The importance of life is about living it however you want to. This will make you successful because it makes you happy.

And happiness, after all, is the closest thing we have to a fountain of youth.

Acknowledgments

I am extremely grateful to have such wonderful friends and family who have supported me in all my endeavours. Working for oneself is one of the loneliest places in the world and I thank you all for being there when needed.

To all the clients I have had the pleasure to train, I can assure you that I have learned as much from you all as you have from me. You have helped me develop my coaching practice to a point I would not have thought possible when I first qualified as a Personal Trainer. I thank you all so very much.

To all the Personal Trainers I have taught. It is an absolute joy to serve such an inspiring profession and I hope I have served you well. Thank you for your support and your efforts in developing an incredible job role.

Finally, to my coach, Tony J Selimi. Tapping into my infinite wisdom is an ongoing process, I know. However, without you I never would have started. I would still be the frustrated, angry, little boy you first met if I hadn't had you to help me see the light that I now know I am.

Thank you all!

Testimonials

"I was recommended to Paul to help me with some lower back pain and what I thought was a lack of flexibility around my hip area. Paul opened my eyes to increasing mobility with some simple exercises and use of a foam roller. After his advice and just one month, my range of hip movement had increased significantly and the back pain is negligible. Paul has modern and innovative ideas on nutrition and fitness, and his personal style is very friendly and easy to work with. Paul is the future of personal training."

GRANT TAYLOR, PARTNER, PERIDOT PARTNERS

"I can safely say that Paul is the best personal trainer that I have ever worked with. He gets the balance right between motivation and fun, and the results achieved have been nothing short of outstanding."

PAUL WEEDON, FOUNDER, RED24 MANAGEMENT

"Working with Paul as my Personal Trainer has changed my whole perspective on training and fitness – all for the better. Over the nine months we worked together Paul ensured I saw real results in the gym. I looked fitter and stronger –. more than that, though, he ensured that change was holistic, and therefore sustainable. We looked at diet and lifestyle. In the gym, the training was more rounded. It wasn't just about lifting bigger weights, it was smarter and more varied than that. And, as a result, I can now lift bigger weights. Significantly though, I also feel better in myself and have more energy."

ANDY COOPER, PARTNER, THINKTANK INTERNATIONAL RESEARCH

"Paul is a motivational trainer, he inspired my wife and me to develop our fitness by personalising a training programme that was time efficient and achievable. This was especially important given our time pressures and busy lives. Results were faster than I anticipated and the methods taught have stuck with us."

MARK PICKERING, FOUNDING DIRECTOR, ARLINGCLOSE TREASURY

"Paul really helped me develop my work/life balance. By focusing on both my nutrition and my fitness it really helped me achieve my goals faster."

ANDREW TOPHAM, CO-FOUNDER & MD, VISION NINE

"As a keen swimmer and surfer, I had started to bulk on weight through training for endurance. This had a knock on effect as I ended up putting on two stone in weight, which acted like a handicap on the hockey pitch. When I decided to lose the weight I struggled through lack of time, managing a small business as well as a young family, which meant lack of time for sleep, good exercise and healthy eating.

I knew that I needed to get myself back on track so that I could have greater energy for work and family. Paul helped me develop a plan that enabled me to manage the key areas of my life without overwhelming what little spare time I now had. I shifted over a stone in two months and have kept it off. Most importantly, with Paul's help I now spend better quality time with my family, eat more healthily and have had my best hockey season ever. Business is booming too!"

ROBIN WAITE, AUTHOR, *ONLINE BUSINESS STARTUP*

"Paul is a great personal trainer. He really helped me with my strength and conditioning. I was having some issues with my knees and he took me through a programme that helped strengthen my legs and allowed me to put more weight on the knees and relieve the pressure. He was great at his job and was always on hand with any additional advice or support. Paul helped me reduce the pain, correct my posture and strengthen my core. I would recommend him to my friends each and every time."

IKE OKOLIE, FOUNDER, ASCENSION LTD

"Paul helped me recover from a lower back injury which plagued me for more than two years. Paul had a close working relationship with my physiotherapist and together they developed a training programme that enabled me to fully recover. The rehab focused mainly on developing my core, and improving the movement around my hips. Following my rehab I was soon competing in my first '10k rat race' at Battersea Power Station! I have 100% confidence in Paul's ability."

SIMON WATSON, FOUNDER, GREENFIELD SOLUTIONS

The Author

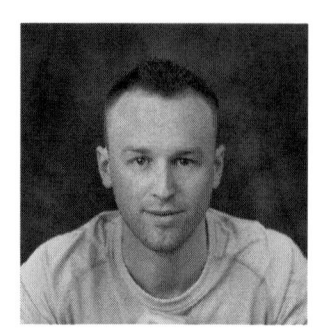

In his time as a Personal Trainer, Paul has worked with over 200 clients, helping them become pain free and feeling energised and youthful once again. In addition to this, Paul has also educated over 300 of the UK's Personal Trainers through courses and customised workshops.

Since entering the health and fitness industry in 2010, Paul has found that virtually all of his clients were experiencing musculoskeletal problems. Having gone through many of these problems himself, Paul knew that he needed to recalibrate and realign his clients before higher intensity training could begin.

Paul also experienced first-hand the pitfalls that business owners fall into as a result of chasing success. This left him low on time, energy, and motivation to look after his health in the best way. Paul is now on a mission to help entrepreneurs overcome physical pain and rebuild their bodies to be robust enough to handle the rigours of business ownership.

Printed in Great Britain
by Amazon.co.uk, Ltd.,
Marston Gate.